WHOLE BODY
MEDITATIONS

Other books by Lorin Roche

Breath Taking

Meditation Secrets for Women

Meditation Made Easy

WHOLE BODY
MEDITATIONS

Igniting Your Natural Instinct to Heal

LORIN ROCHE, PH.D.

RODALE

Printed in the United States of America
Rodale Inc. makes every effort to use acid-free (∞), recycled paper ♺.

Cover Designer: Christopher Rhoads
Interior Designer: Jeff Puda
Illustrator: Greg Couch

Library of Congress Cataloging-in-Publication Data

    Roche, Lorin.
    Whole body meditations : igniting your natural instinct to heal / Lorin Roche.
        p.   cm.
    Includes index.
    ISBN 1–57954–345–6 paperback
    1. Meditation.   2. Healing—Religious aspects.   I. Title.
    BL627 .R615   2002
    158.1'2—dc21   2001007023

Distributed to the book trade by St. Martin's Press
2 4 6 8 10 9 7 5 3 1   paperback

Visit us on the Web at www.rodalestore.com, or call us toll-free at (800) 848-4735.

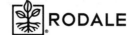

RODALE

WE **INSPIRE** AND **ENABLE** PEOPLE TO IMPROVE
THEIR LIVES AND THE WORLD AROUND THEM

Neither [medicine nor surgery] can do anything

but remove obstructions; neither can cure;

nature alone cures. . . . Nature heals the wound. . . .

[W]hat Nursing has to do in either case, is to put the patient

in the best condition for nature to act upon him.

—Florence Nightingale

Contents

Introduction ✳ **ix**

CHAPTER 1 The Quest for Wholeness ✳**3**

CHAPTER 2 The Instinct to Heal ✳**59**

CHAPTER 3 Meditation as Healing Attention ✳**109**

CHAPTER 4 The Whole Body Scan ✳**179**

Sources, Resources, and Further Explorations ✳**221**

Index ✳**231**

Introduction

Human beings are born with a great capacity for self-healing. As we move through our lives, this healing and repair function works continuously and spontaneously, especially when we rest. The mind-body system tends to heal itself of whatever injuries it has suffered, whether they be emotional, physical, or mental, whether it be simple daily fatigue or deeper trauma. Sometimes it takes longer than we would like to return to a sense of wellness; sometimes the attention of an external healer is required; and at times we are left with some scars. The rhythm of life is that we go forth boldly and live, and then we repair to our nest and rest up in order to do it all again. The more quickly and thoroughly we can revive and heal, the sooner we can get back to doing what we love.

For thousands of years and in many cultures, wise women and men have practiced daily meditation as a way of cooperating with the body's inner healing wisdom and living life in a more continually rejuvenated state. In the latter part of the 20th century, as medical instruments evolved, scientists began to be interested in measuring the physiological changes evoked by meditation. Over decades, researchers in many labs have found that indeed, meditation seems to boost health in general and contributes measurably to the management and healing of many ailments: addictions, allergies, anxiety, arthritis, asthma, back pain, cancer, carpal tunnel syndrome, chronic fatigue, eating disorders, gastrointestinal problems, headaches, immune system disorders, heart disease, hypertension, infertility, insomnia, menopause, muscle tension, skin problems, and tinnitus.

Again and again in different studies, researchers have found that meditation often aids significantly in treating symptoms, preventing relapses, and helping the body to heal itself. Also, meditation is something that the patient can do on his or her own, at home—and it's free. For all these reasons, self-help groups and 12-step programs for people with all kinds of ailments often employ meditation as one of their tools for coping. Meditation is something the body and mind naturally want to do, and it has been found that anyone who wants to can meditate, with a little bit of instruction.

How can one simple practice, in which a person sits for half an hour with the eyes closed, thinking of something pleasant, produce all these diverse benefits? It turns out that when you meditate, within several minutes the body becomes more restful than in deep sleep and the muscles become very relaxed, yet you are awake and alert inside. These conditions allow the nerves and the body to let go of stress and fatigue. The relaxation and sense of ease carry over for hours after meditation, contributing to a more centered and healthy approach to life. Doctors have known for decades that human illness is stress related, meaning that chronic stress is a significant factor in making existing medical conditions worse, causing flare-ups, and in general taxing the overall health of an individual. And the list of stress-related illnesses known to medical science is very similar to the list of ailments detailed above.

When scientists have tested meditators, they have found that within a couple of minutes their instruments detect a whole set of physiologic changes: metabolic rate, blood pressure, heart rate, muscle tension, and stress hormones circulating in the blood all decrease. This is the mirror opposite of what happens when we are scared or stressed; in the stress response all those indexes increase. It makes sense then that meditation is a good way of helping the body restore itself from the wear and tear caused by stress.

During meditation, even though overall there is a great deal of relaxation and repose, the brain is very busy. The paradox is, you can't relax without letting go of tension, and in letting go of tension you remember all the things you were tense about. Whatever thoughts, sensations, or emotions you have been holding at bay by staying tense are free to flood your awareness and be dealt with. Meditation is a highly alert state, and so you often find yourself shifting every few seconds between delicious rest and anxiety, until your system works out just the right balance between ease, excitement, and alarm to handle the various challenges of your life, including all your relationships and even any medical conditions.

Meditation is definitely not a monotonous state of inner blankness. Even though everyone wants the brain to shut up during meditation, it almost never happens. Rather, meditation is a dynamic condition of relaxation and tension, inner peacefulness and excited musings about work and love. When I ask people who have quit meditating why they stopped, the most common response is, "I just couldn't get into it. I couldn't make my mind blank." They admit that yes, they felt relaxation, and yes, they felt better afterward, but all that inner noise—that can't be right. Almost universally, people blame themselves because their brains are so busy.

This play of opposites that occurs constantly in meditation reminds me of the way vaccinations work. When you get a vaccination, you take into your body a weakened form of a virus or bacteria. Often the vaccine is just a portion of the structure of the pathogen, enough to give the immune system a pattern to recognize and stimulate the production of antibodies. In meditation, what the mind-body system does instinctively is to enter a state of safety and relaxation and then replay portions and fragments of stressors, so that it can generate a more elegant and adaptive response. So you find yourself becoming very involved with memories of times you were startled, snatches of conversations, the sense memory of muscular tension, and all the other aspects of what you feel emotionally and physically when stressed. This happens whether you want it to or not, for it's an aspect of the body's adaptation and spontaneous self-healing. To the extent that you have a rich and full life, your brain is going to be very busy in meditation.

If you don't understand the rhythms of meditation and become intimate with how this dynamic feels in your own body, then you will tend to resist it, just as children hate getting vaccinations. You may mistakenly think, "This isn't helping; it's just making me worse." And, truth be told, it's easy to feel that way. I once had a whole series of vaccinations as preparation for traveling in equatorial Africa, and some of them made me feverish for days. But it's a hell of a lot better than getting the full-blown disease. It's better to pull out the thorns than leave them to fester. And it's better to give your body a chance to work out a more elegant way of dealing with stressors, rather than stay in the alarm response for long periods of time.

You can see from this description that meditation is not one state but rather a continually changing inner theater of quiet intensity, in which each breath brings new drama, catharsis, rebirth—and yes, healing. From the time you close your eyes to the time you open them 20 minutes later, you have gone through an entire odyssey of the heart, mind, body, and sometimes spirit. Within that time, many minute-long adventure cycles occur in which you go from feeling totally at ease, to immersion in a daydream concerning your greatest life challenges, to relaxation again.

Meditation feels different each time you do it, and each moment of meditation is different from the next as your body rests up, revitalizes itself, and tunes itself for action. The more you cooperate with this process, the more the vaccination quality becomes specific to you and whatever stresses you are facing, whether they be of long hours, your aches and pains, too many tasks to juggle, or a medical condition you are suffering from. If you find your way through to actually meditating every day, you will soon realize that this is the deepest quality of rest you have ever had in your life, and as your body gets used to it, you will feel yourself healing very gently and gradually, on a deep level. Whatever you are suffering from or in pain about, whether it be emotional or physical, will call your attention and will become the focus of your healing meditation for a while.

The beneficial effects of meditation have been widely publicized, and consequently millions of people throughout the world have been experimenting with the practice. There are how-to books available in many languages, and the instructions for effective meditation are quite simple: Sit somewhere safe, close your eyes, and attend restfully to a focus. As a focus, you can select anything you love to pay attention to, whether it be an image in nature, the rhythm of your own breathing, or the memory of a melody. When your mind wanders, which it will, gently return to the focus. Continue in this way for 20 minutes or so, then go about your day.

What has been happening, though, is that most people who begin meditation quit in frustration within a few days or weeks. The follow-through rate is much higher when the student is working directly with a meditation teacher or a therapist, doctor, or yoga teacher, but only a small percentage of the people who want to use meditation have access to a teacher or guide. This book is written to offer useful information to that other 90 percent of the aspiring meditators, who want to meditate on their own, without a teacher, as part of their general self-care.

❧

I have found that people who are hurting in some way have a natural affinity for meditation. Illness disrupts our lives, and the symptoms often make us feel like resting, and we seek out healing. In researching this book, I spoke with people suffering from all the stress-related ailments mentioned above, who are using meditation to help manage their illness. My original plan was to get a sense of what techniques are best for each ailment, but what I heard was that healing is an individual thing. It struck me that it was important to develop an approach to meditation to suit the person, not the disease.

I asked people, "What works? What works for you, in your situation?" Many people told me something along the lines of, "What works for me is nature: fresh air, sunlight, the earth, water, rivers, the ocean. I meditate on that if I'm inside, and I often go outside to meditate. I am often in a building, but when I close my eyes to meditate I breathe as if I am standing on my favorite mountain or beach, looking out over infinity." And further, "Yes, there are techniques, but the important thing is to find what you love, what makes you want to be well, what reminds you of when you were well, and meditate with that. Be with that, and that's the technique." As a consequence, instead of writing about specific ailments and meditation techniques, I found myself writing about nature, the elements, the instincts, and the rhythm of adventure. Your body is the closest bit of nature to you. Perceive it as nature—as made up of the elements and instincts.

❧

The point of any good meditation book is to be an ally on your journeys in your inner world. You do not need to know everything in this book in order to meditate—you may need to know just one bit of information, represented by one sentence, paragraph, or chapter. Since meditation is an instinctive skill that is built in to human beings, we do not so much learn it as learn to allow it to happen. The skill of meditation is in cooperating with what life is doing on every level of your being—biological, relational, and spiritual. You have the skills of meditation within you already because meditation involves being open to your senses and following your instincts. Tolerating this openness is one of the major challenges along the path of meditation.

In adapting to your life thus far, you may have learned to shut down some of your senses and block some of your instincts. In that case, your path may involve unlearning as a preliminary step, because meditation works best when all your senses and instincts have free play.

The approach to meditation I recommend is quite simple: Just accept every impulse that you witness in meditation as a healing impulse. In every moment, the brain, nervous system, mind, body, and heart are working to heal themselves. Every part is working to fulfill its relationship to the whole. The mind is extremely purposeful, and every impulse you perceive going through you when you are meditating has a deep connection to life. If you follow it, it will take you deep into life's essence.

There is a sequence of little skills you need to learn within the first few minutes and days of beginning to meditate that have to do with accepting the range and fluctuating quality of your experience. In those first few seconds, minutes, and days of meditation you will learn one way or the other of dealing with emotions, sensations, and the many kinds of thoughts that arise. These first few moments of meditation are a new beginning and an opportunity to make a completely new deal with your life, a fresh approach.

The essence of meditation is to select something you love, that you adore, and then be with it, rest with it, and see what happens. Something profound happens when you sit there and let your love impact you deeply and transform you from the inside. Meditation is being there and noticing all the nuances as love arises in you, changes your breathing, alters the way your heart beats, changes your thinking, and lights up your senses.

Make a connection between the act of reading and closing your eyes to meditate. Every few paragraphs or pages, or whenever you find something interesting, look at the horizon or close your eyes and breathe with the thought and the feeling behind it. Let your mind drift. Or get up and take a walk and mull it over. Your real teacher is the interaction between your attention and what you love. Turn and return always to that.

WHOLE BODY
MEDITATIONS

The Quest for Wholeness

Nature wants you to be whole and intact, as healthy as you can be. When your body can't easily heal some injury on its own, it sends you signals—aches, pains, or other sensations—that it needs help. If you are experiencing persistent pain or distress, you may have to go on a quest—a healing quest for wholeness.

This is the fundamental rhythm of life: sensing a need, addressing that need, then moving on to the next one. The rhythm of sensing a need, paying attention to it, finding a way to satisfy it, is something life is continually engaged in on every level—each cell, each organ, each area of the body, each instinct, every aspect of your heart and mind, are engaged in the rhythm. Some cycles take place in a minute, as in getting a glass of water. Some take years, as in finding a mate, the right place to live, or the ideal job. Some take seconds. In meditation, you feel all these rhythms simultaneously, and your experience is primarily made up of the music of these intersecting rhythms, which play out in seconds, minutes, hours, days, weeks, and months. You experience this pattern in practical matters such as the search for a home and job. You need one; you look for one; and when you find one, you do what you can to keep it. You also experience this dynamic when you feel the urge for and seek out fulfillment in the sexual, spiritual, and emotional realms. When it is healing that you need, it's the knowledge inherent in your own body that you should rely on to guide you through the process. Meditation can help you access this self-knowledge so that you may recover more quickly and completely.

Wellness is a whole body experience. It means that you feel alive to all your capabilities and talents and relate to life through them. Sometimes we can feel as if we once were whole but no longer are, as if something has been lost along the way. You may think, *I don't feel at home in myself anymore.* Maybe you have partly gotten over an injury or a betrayal but in the process have lost your zest for living. Or you may feel that deep healing is something you hunger for but have never experienced.

This hunger is like a nutritional need. Our bodies and psyches are attuned to this craving and they call on us to satisfy it. But it's up to us to fully investigate these callings to find out what we lack, check it against our past experiences, and experiment with what might work to heal us. Again, meditation can help.

HELP HEAL YOURSELF

Although meditation is an overall, whole body response, it does have measurable effects on specific parts of the body. Meditation has been shown to be effective in helping reduce symptoms or speed healing of many ailments, particularly those caused by or made worse by stress, including:

Allergies	Gastrointestinal problems	Muscle tension
Anxiety	HIV+/AIDS	Palpitations
Arthritis	Headaches, migraine and others	Perimenopause/ menopause
Asthma		
Back pain	Heart disease	Rashes and other skin problems
Cancer	Hypertension	
Carpal tunnel syndrome	Infertility	Shortness of breath
Chronic fatigue syndrome	Insomnia and other sleep disorders	Tinnitus
		Temporomandibular joint disease
Chronic pain	Joint pain	

In addition, meditation is used as part of programs that treat:

Addiction	Eating disorders	Preparation for surgery
Depression	Lupus	Sexual dysfunction
Dizziness		

It is characteristic of meditation that the beneficial effects do not fade with time; rather, benefits get stronger over time in people who start meditating in order to deal with some particular ailment and keep on meditating after their initial success.

The quest for wholeness can feel like—and be seen as—a mythic journey. You have to leave your familiar sense of yourself and wander into the unknown. In fairy tales and myths, there is always something amiss in the kingdom or queendom; otherwise, there would be no story. The crops are wilting. The king is sick. A daughter is being held captive. The hero, who is sometimes noble and valiant and at other times a bum-

THE MYTHIC CYCLE

The mythic cycle is evident in even the most basic and mundane life functions. Any desire, the movement toward satisfying it, and the act of receiving fulfillment reflects the dynamics of the quest.

In the following example, the body's need for water leads to a journey that ends in a successful resolution, the healing or quenching of the thirst.

1. **The call**—*I am thirsty.*

2. **Refusing the call**—*I'll get a drink later; I'm busy.*

3. **Crossing the threshold**—The need gets stronger until it can't be ignored. *Okay, okay, I'll get something to drink.*

4. **Facing obstacles**—*Damn! I don't have enough change for the machine.*

5. **Enlisting helpers**—"Thanks, Donna, I'll pay you back after lunch."

6. **Reaching for the elixir**—*Ahhhhh, water! Life-giving, sweet-tasting water!* (Or cola, or coffee, or juice—your elixir of choice.)

7. **The journey home**—You return to your desk feeling satisfied—until the next time. *Now where was I . . .*

bling fool, seeks out the secret path through to the underworld and there obtains the key to success or, for our use, to self-healing.

Survivors of serious diseases often say they feel like they've been on an odyssey through the health care system. The right doctor can be hard to find, difficult to get a timely appointment with, prohibitively expensive, or a long distance away. Many unhelpful physicians may have been contacted, who did not have the time or the inclination to study the case. All of these are good reasons to tap into the full healing force of nature yourself to achieve the wholeness you desire.

Meditation has evolved out of the healing and self-repairing function of the body. The meditative state is one in which the body can access its patterns of wholeness and health, and work to re-create them. This is why when you meditate, you become aware of whatever you need to complete yourself.

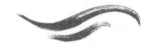

Healing and Wholeness

Meditation gives you direct and powerful access to your healing wisdom. When we meditate, we release ourselves into the body's template of health, which is a whole-body state of flow and balance. Your entire nervous system longs to reunite with that, and takes advantage of the meditation time to bathe in this sense of wholeness and

The Journey to Health

In terms of dealing with health problems, the mythic journey may look something like this:

- First, you have a feeling that something may be wrong: the call. There is an ache, a signal from your body.
- You brush the pain aside, ignore the signal, refuse the call.
- But the pain is still there the next day, or it comes back before long. Your symptoms get progressively harder to ignore.
- You start gathering information about indicated ailments by reading or talking to others.
- You call your family doctor or hunt down a specialist, schedule an appointment, and wait.
- Now you're in the waiting room at the doctor's.
- You finally meet with the doctor and communicate your symptoms.
- You monitor the doctor's body language and manner. You wonder, "Is this the physician for me? Do I trust him?"
- You listen closely to the results of the exam and the doctor's diagnosis.
- You may seek a second opinion and then have to sort out the confusion caused by different diagnoses, healing modalities (conventional versus alternative), and suggested remedies.

deal with any obstacles to experiencing wholeness. Meditation in fact is the technique of intentionally giving in to the body's innate motion toward healing and wholeness.

The first step toward whole body healing is to learn to cooperate with nature, the wisdom that has evolved in you, in the human body, over the ages. Meditation is a

◆ You follow the regimen the doctor or naturopath prescribes.

◆ You deal with the high cost of paying for the treatment and the time involved.

◆ You prepare for surgery, if that is indicated. You develop a rapport with the anesthesiologist, and afterward, reorient yourself.

◆ You cooperate as best you can with the healing process.

◆ You may have to accept and enact drastic changes in lifestyle, learn to live with physical limitations or an ongoing medication or rehab program, or maybe even face the fact that you're dying.

◆ In any case, you must recover a healthy attitude and emerge into the world looking to be whole again.

Meditation can help with each stage of this journey. Each step has its own tricky negotiations. For example, it can be very comforting when a physician dismisses your symptoms as normal aches and pains; the relief is immediate. But then you have to decide for yourself if the doctor really listened to your concerns rather than just brushing you off. Did he consider your complaint from every angle, or is he just thinking of getting through the other eight patients he has to see in the next hour? Meditating gives you clarity— access to clear signals from your body and a clear mind to decide how to proceed.

natural state, part of the body's survival strategy, and as such the body knows what to do to come into the balance that it craves. The interplay of your body, your nervous system, and awareness generates the experience of many different impulses—sensations, emotions, thoughts, and desires. Cooperating with nature means allowing these impulses to flow through you and inform you. You learn to follow their lead into your-self, your self, and into health. This is both the simplest and the hardest part of med-itation. Simple because the impulses come up whether you want them to or not. Hard because these impulses feel wild, infinitely varied, and nonmeditative, and you have to learn to not control your thoughts and feelings in any way but simply witness them with great tenderness and respect.

Illness often leads us to mistrust the body because it seems defective, and so we try to ignore the signals; or we treat the symptoms instead of the underlying cause of whatever malady we may be suffering from. To help make ourselves well, we need to learn to trust ourselves and to listen closely so that we can reinhabit our bodies.

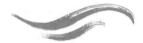

Reinhabiting the Body

Everyday stress, such as being late, hurried, worried, or overworked, tends to chase us out of our bodies. We all have experienced this many times in rushing to get some-where but mentally arriving quite a bit after our bodies get there. To an even greater extent, physical or emotional trauma and the pain they cause also incite us to disso-ciate from our bodies. We don't want to be in there to *feel*. This can be helpful, as the shock and denial may allow us to survive until we can get to a safe place, or until we realize that the place where we are is safe enough—then the healing can begin. Sometimes, though, we never make it to that safe place. Yet we crave to return there, to return to ourselves. If we don't reinhabit the body through a practice such as meditation, we may find ourselves craving drugs, food, or destructive behaviors. No one would take cocaine or heroin unless they were in anguish.

When we abandon the body or parts of the body, we usually do not notice it at the time. We tend to try to put off dealing with the fact of our injury. It's like feeling the first pangs of thirst and brushing it off: *I can wait—I'm not that thirsty.* But pain is a calling that gets harder to resist. In meditation, we stop trying to get away from the pain and instead allow attention to be with the sensations, motions, and emotions underlying the pain. When we do this, the natural healing instincts of the body are free to work. When we do the opposite, when we stay overly busy and distract ourselves in

VISUALIZE THE JOURNEY

Once you understand that meditation is like a mythic journey, with allies and obstacles and a continually changing path of adventure, you can be more at home with it. Examine the past course of your quest for wholeness. Imagine what the road ahead might be like, and look for parallel experiences in novels, operas, musicals, movies, sitcoms, comic books, and magazine stories. Notice how the conflicts and resolutions that are played out, and even the imagery that commonly appears in the popular media, are similar to those that show up on the screen of your mind during meditation.

order to avoid feeling the pain, we can postpone our healing, at least for a while. I know quite a few people who create little emergencies for themselves on a regular basis in order to limit their quiet time.

First of all, pain motivates us to get out of a bad situation. Then it prompts us to care for ourselves and tend to our wounds. When you meditate, you become aware of many little imbalances and discomforts, and simply paying attention to them lets the body engage in rebalancing itself. This almost always hurts, and in various ways. Sometimes it's as if your own body is scolding you for abusing it, like the painful protest of sore muscles when you finally sit down after a workout. If you persevere through the sensations, they tend to turn into great relief and pleasure.

When you are in the process of reinhabiting your body, you will encounter obstacles and allies in the form of painful and pleasurable sensations and your responses to them. As you come into your body, you begin to feel everything that previously, out of fear, you were avoiding—even the good things. It is only when you come down off the stress response that you feel these good feelings. Reinhabiting the body means getting used to this rich world of ever-changing sensations.

The process is similar to what you feel when you have been sitting and your legs or feet "fall asleep." When you uncross your legs and restore circulation, you feel uncomfortable tinglings as the nerves wake up. Restoring free circulation of all your life energies is the goal—the promised elixir—of whole body meditation. Sometimes this waking-up process is joyful, and sometimes you have to face very uncomfortable sensations. The difference between cutting off circulation to your legs and what happens in meditation is that the process is usually much more gradual. It was over a period of years that you developed your personality and out of some necessity cut yourself off from your full being. And it is over years that the circulation will be restored.

The demons, monsters, and dragons you need to confront in the process are your own life energies that you have been ignoring. This is the hell you have to pay when you want to reenter the body: You have to pay attention to these demons and convert them back into your own life force to make them available for love, work, and play.

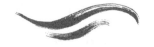

Initiation to the Self

Any quest involves initiations and rites of passage, and the quest for wholeness is no exception. It is common in cultures around the world for initiations to involve pain or suffering and seemingly insurmountable challenges. The initiate has to find resources within herself that she did not know she had. Sometimes, she is put to a life-or-death test.

Naturally, we are changed by such an ordeal. One of the healing challenges is to accept this changed status as a gift. Veiled inside of every discomfort, every healing crisis, is opportunity. It can happen with a toothache, a broken bone, or a chronic disease; the gift may be the support of a loved one or simply a renewed appreciation of life and gratitude for health.

When you are dealing with illness or injury, you have to face the fear and challenge of being at the mercy of forces greater than yourself. Your initiation is to find the inner resources that allow you to pass through to a new level of being. Your task is to create a world—an internal and external environment—in which you can thrive. You do this by answering the call and attending the instincts you are neglecting. This is your internal medicine. This is the elixir you are seeking.

You may be lacking sufficient attention to only one of your instincts—self-nurturing, aggression, rest, play—but the lack of that element can be holding back your healing. For want of the natural chemicals released by your body in response to that element or instinct, you are being starved of something.

Although we may crave what we are missing, we are also terrified of it. Just ask

A WALK ON THE WILD SIDE

The call of meditation is a call of the wild, the serene inner wilds. You are called on to engage the natural forces of your being more directly. Of course, wilderness is paradoxical. If you have ever been to the desert, stood in the middle of a vast forest, or walked alone on a deserted stretch of beach, you know there is nothing like the deep sense of peace. And yet, because it is nature, all around you the insects, plants, and animals are hunting one another.

someone who is a nice person, giving and friendly, what it feels like to reclaim their aggression, their killer instinct. It may feel to them like a fate worse than death, a descent into hell, to activate their anger. Or ask someone who is not used to what it feels like to open up emotionally and surrender to another person. Many men would rather die than open their hearts; and many do.

There is probably no one who has not left some part of himself behind. Lots of mothers I know were once hellions, raising a ruckus when they were in high school or college. Then over the decades they lost touch with that lively rebelliousness. Often the call back into liveliness comes in the form of their rebellious daughters or sons. They have to access that earlier part of themselves to be able to skillfully handle the situation. The same is true for fathers, and both men and women lose important parts of themselves in adapting to the workplace and becoming professionally successful. They may have lost their ability to relax, to love, or to gaze into another person's eyes without looking for weakness. Reconnecting with their former selves through whole body meditation is a powerful way to initiate a new, healthier pattern of behavior.

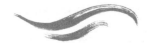

The Healing Cycle

The journey into the body replicates the structure of the mythic cycle, in which we are called to depart from everyday life, encounter obstacles, enlist allies in our search for the elixir—and then return to our normal lives. Like the mythic cycle, the healing cycle has similar distinct stages: the call, the refusal of the call, threshold crossing, initiation, finding the elixir, and bringing it home.

SYMPTOMS AS CALLINGS

Symptoms are messengers delivering word that something in the kingdom of your body is amiss. They are signals that call your attention to an imbalance or injury so that you can cooperate with your own healing process. You can use meditation to both hear and answer the call.

When you feel pain or stress, there are two essential responses: You can dissociate and attempt to get on with life, or you can associate and cooperate. Hearing the call involves allowing attention to be drawn to the uncomfortable sensations; in other words, you feel the pain. The temptation is to try not to feel it, to try to make it go away without getting the message. But if you don't hear the call, you won't get the message, and your body will suffer until you do. It will also continue to call you, ever more loudly, to get your attention.

Answering the call involves cooperating with your body to facilitate healing. Sometimes our quest for wholeness needs to be directed outward—we need to go out and find a doctor or therapist and undergo a treatment or take a drug. Sometimes the quest is properly directed inward—we need to go to a place within ourselves where we can heal. In either case, we need to find the missing

THE RHYTHM OF THE HEALING QUEST

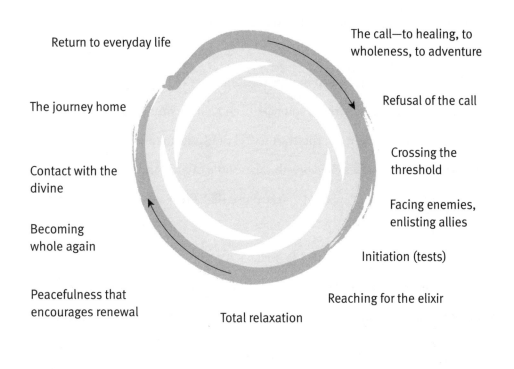

Return to everyday life

The call—to healing, to wholeness, to adventure

The journey home

Refusal of the call

Contact with the divine

Crossing the threshold

Becoming whole again

Facing enemies, enlisting allies

Initiation (tests)

Peacefulness that encourages renewal

Reaching for the elixir

Total relaxation

element, the neglected instinct that can naturally help restore wholeness.

Notice the way a symptom drives you to attend to your body. Have you ever found out what a symptom wants and given it to yourself? I'll bet you have. Perhaps the symptom is the craving for alcohol. Grab the meaning of the symptom—an attempt to induce relaxation—and give it to yourself directly. Oddly enough, this may feel like theft. You are stealing back the power that alcohol, magic foods, or other escapist rituals have had over you in the past and reclaiming this power for yourself. On the mythic quest for the elixir, sometimes it has to be stolen.

The rhythm of the quest can involve the longer arc of a healing journey, or it can play out in a few seconds. Perhaps you have been holding your breath because you are tense. For lack of sufficient air, you start to feel tired and anxious. You sense the need to do something, and take a deep breath. These little callings and their fulfillments become obvious when you meditate. You sense that every few seconds is an entire odyssey.

As you go through your daily life, make it a point to listen for seemingly minor callings—a bit of stiffness in your joints or muscles—and explore what happens if you answer them by stretching, breathing deeply, or relaxing in the moment. You may just feel like you've downed a quick draft of precious elixir.

REFUSING THE CALL

Because hearing and then answering the call to heal involves feeling our pain and overcoming obstacles, it's understandable that our initial response might be to refuse the call. Ways of refusing the call include deliberately setting off in the wrong direction or dragging your baggage with you when you should take only what you can easily carry. Or you might refuse to face whatever immediately comes up to be dealt with.

Jung said somewhere that the purpose of therapy is to extricate yourself from your inauthentic suffering, which is a distraction, and engage with your real suffering, your authentic anguish over life. What happens very often in meditation is that the authentic suffering comes up immediately and we turn away from it and make meditation itself the obstacle. For example, we distract ourselves from the pain of having a closed heart by focusing on how the noise of kids playing is ruining our focus. In meditation, the rules are simple: Let attention go where it is called. Sometimes sensations call our attention, sometimes they command memories or thoughts.

Even if a student hears me say, "Don't resist thoughts," and nods her head, a minute later, in the midst of meditation, she might start trying to push out thoughts. I can tell by the furrowed brow and the stern scowl. This situation of trying to block out thoughts may result in her blocking out the very call to meditate, or stalemating the process. Refusing to let thoughts tell you what they have to say is like covering your ears and screaming "Yada yada yada . . ." when the mysterious guide who has arrived to call you on the quest is attempting to tell you in which direction to set off.

Crossing Thresholds

We encounter a threshold whenever we experience or are asked to experience more of something than we are used to. In daily life, there are many thresholds we come up against: how many hours we can work, how steadfastly we can concentrate on the

(continued on page 24)

LORIN'S NOTEBOOK

PHYLLIS: REFUSING THE CALL

Phyllis was an attractive woman in her late forties. Her children had gone off to college, and now that she had an empty nest she finally felt that she had time for herself. During her first session, she slipped into meditation very easily. I usually have people meditate for brief periods: a minute, then 2 minutes, then 3, then 5. I have them meditate longer only when they can handle the shorter stretches without straining. When Phyllis opened her eyes after each of the first three meditations, it was as if she were coming back from a long way away. After her 3-minute meditation, I asked her to look out the window at the garden and tell me what she saw. She described seeing the light on the leaves as seemingly magical, enchanting, appearing in Technicolor. Her whole body seemed suffused with pleasure.

We were a minute into her 5-minute meditation when she started frowning a bit. I asked her to open her eyes and tell me what she was experiencing.

"Well, I was all relaxed and these thoughts started bothering me, so I was trying to shoo them away."

"Thoughts aren't flies, even though they seem to buzz around," I said. I asked her what sorts of thoughts she was having.

"Painful memories." The situation, I gathered, went something like this: There had been a period long ago when Phyllis was very involved in the kids' lives. She and her husband weren't having sex and she thought he was fine with it. She was fulfilled as a mother and very, very busy. She found out years later that he had been having an affair with a woman down the street whom she knew slightly. The painful memories she didn't want to see were horrid images of the woman looking at her smugly, the woman looking trim and happy, the woman at parties in her house. Now, bothered by those memories, she found herself wondering if her husband had bought the woman a certain dress.

"Those kinds of thoughts come up to be healed," I explained. "What's happening is that you are relaxed and your guard is down. Your body has decided to bring up something that pains you deeply so that in the safety of meditation those feelings can be faced. These are powerful feelings, and they have gotten lodged in your emotional body. It takes a lot of energy and tension to keep from feeling such emotions."

As I was saying all of this, tears came to her eyes, but then she angrily set her face in an expression that said "I can't" or "I won't." At this point Phyllis and I were at an impasse. Or rather, Phyllis and meditation were. Her lifelong strategy had been to not let dark thoughts get to her, to keep her house clean and days busy so she could avoid getting depressed. This was a great talent, and it certainly got her through a whole phase of her life, but at the expense of blocking much of her emotions.

I made up a metaphor for her about how sometimes in meditation you have to get down on your hands and knees and scrub. "There you are in all this dirt and grunge, but it's okay, you are wearing your old clothes, you can take a shower later, and then you will feel really good that a difficult chore is done." I tried to sound as much as I could like an old, wise grandmother. "It's not all looking at the beautiful flowers, dear. Think about what awful stinky stuff compost is made of!"

This was the time in life for Phyllis to explore herself, but her habit was to close the door on many rooms of her inner house because they seemed creepy,

(continued)

LORIN'S NOTEBOOK (CONT.)

full of yucky things, old memories, anger. She was hoping that meditation would act like Valium, a tranquilizer that would let her keep on leading a cheery life though her nest was empty and didn't provide ample distraction from the pain.

Phyllis isn't wrong—meditation can be a pretty good Valium substitute, and a person in her position probably can avoid a lot of difficult inner confrontations for years. But if she would have let the painful memories surface and just cry during meditation, or shake with anger, she would most likely have felt fantastic afterward. Cleansed.

Phyllis didn't want to go way back into the past and invent misery for herself. She didn't want to stay angry at her husband and fight about the affair. She didn't want to be a victim. She wanted to keep it together, have a good time in life, and take a lot of trips.

The problem with this approach is that Phyllis was like a person with a wound, and when the doctor—in this case the healing meditation—touched it with antiseptic, she batted away his arm and said, "Ow, you're hurting me," and that was that. In meditation, the relaxation she had experienced brought her into contact with her hurt, and the two coexisted for a while. Even though it seemed to Phyllis that the thoughts were ruining her meditation, in truth that's the perfect situation for healing. The painful memories were a sign of success, that she was relaxed enough to admit to consciousness what was really, deeply bothering her.

You could say that Phyllis had refused the call of her inner life. You could say she wanted to dictate exactly how her healing should proceed. You could say she was torn between impulses and needed time to negotiate how she was going to satisfy these voices pulling her in different directions. In the first 20 minutes of her first meditation session, Phyllis went through all of this, and in this she is not unusual. It often happens that the goal of one's healing quest becomes clear just a few minutes after beginning meditation. You decide right then whether to trust the process or not. Phyllis never came back for a second session, so I don't know how things turned out for her.

People who have experienced situations like Phyllis's tend to become depressed at some point. The dark thoughts they have been blocking out so zealously finally wear them down, and in their depressed state they do some emotional processing of those awful feelings. You never know, though. At some point Phyllis may have had a really bad day or week and just like that gotten over her anger. Sometimes we "get" things a month, 6 months, or even years later that we can't understand or won't accept on one particular day. Phyllis may have been searching for a better context in which to let go.

This leads us back to the simplicity of one of the basic instructions for meditating: When thoughts come, do not try to block them out. Phyllis could have decided to answer the call then and there and end her quest for wholeness. I bring this up so that you will be prepared to face what occurs during meditation and how rapidly experience changes. You never know from moment to moment what you will experience, but rarely is meditation like taking a number and then waiting years for an appointment with the healer. The calling you have been feeling in your heart to do something for yourself has already done the arranging. Just walk in.

tasks at hand, how many activities we can attend with our kids, how much responsibility we can handle. Crossing such thresholds is not always unpleasant. Think of how intensely pleasurable it would be to give more love or appreciation than you thought yourself capable of. And yet, the thought or act of crossing a threshold—even when love and happiness are on the other side—can be terrifying.

On any quest for wholeness, you may have to cross several thresholds—you may have to decline a certain project at work, admit to a friend that you feel like a failure, or take a long-delayed vacation (don't laugh—some people are very seriously afraid of what might happen if they took an extended vacation). If you are facing a medical problem, you may have to go see a doctor, confess how much you hurt, let yourself be probed, submit to tests, read about illnesses, make hard decisions about which treatment is less horrible, join a support group, take medications, and more. Each one of these activities constitutes a threshold. Most people I know don't like to do such things unless they really, really have to.

A threshold crossing is a good time to access your instincts. Each instinct is a gateway to the inner self and, as such, an aid to navigating the outer world (see "Instincts Lead the Way" on page 66). Any instincts that you avoid can act as obstacles to healing, and this needs to be addressed. For example, if you normally don't get enough rest, you will have to do that; if you don't usually stand up for your point of view, that's what you will have to do. Here again, meditation can help.

When answering the call involves meditating, you are taken across a perceptual threshold. You physically stay in one place, and yet you journey because your view of the world changes as you face new sensations and realizations. If you are seriously ill, you may accept in a deep way the fact that you could die or rather *will* die someday. But even facing lesser hurts and heartbreaks, in meditation you become unusually sensitive to your body, and thoughts zoom everywhere as you release them from control. In this heightened state, healing takes place. That's the time to tackle the big taboos that by habit we shy away from (see "Common Taboos You'll Face on the Quest" on page 37). Once you get used to breaking taboos, it's quite entertaining.

Also, allies tend to show up when we cross thresholds; we meet people who have made positive changes in their own lives and who serve in one way or another to cheer us on. Yes, there will be those who resist change and want you to stay the same, but there will always be someone somewhere who endorses the person you are becoming.

INITIATION

Initiation means to begin, to launch ourselves into a new state of being. The challenge is to accept, to say yes to that different sense of self. Whenever you close your eyes to meditate, within moments you may find yourself being pulled in many different directions as you become aware of how rapidly your brain is working. There is a moment of panic, and the impulse to try to hold on to something, to hold the world together. You feel more like you are being dismembered than being put back together, but that's the process. You have to breathe out before you can breathe in again. You have to let go and fall asleep before you can wake up refreshed. The best way out of this scary situation is to cultivate a sense of safety in the process itself.

One of the reflexes almost everyone has when starting to meditate is to try to slow down the speed of thoughts, but this will only throw you off balance. The thoughts themselves are not the problem; the attempt to control thoughts or feelings is the obstacle. You are presented with a choice when you begin meditating: If you truly want to achieve a restful and renewing state, let your brain think whatever it wants to think, do what it needs to do, without interfering. To the extent that you resist your thoughts, even a tiny bit, meditation will not be as restful and it won't be as healing.

When you meditate, thoughts and feelings take on an enhanced clarity and intensity, and they may change rapidly and in unpredictable ways. A sensation you thought was pain and blocked out now appears to be an emotion of great joy; the fatigue you felt in your legs now seems like a happy sense of being used. Again and again you will find that you need to accept any pain before you can release it. The greater the pain you are in, the more your body will need to release that pain through whatever process it selects: crying, shaking, angry thoughts, falling asleep, a burst of energy, creativity, or just a slow, careful tending until every last hurt has been felt through.

I have worked with many people who cried during every meditation for months before finally emerging renewed and feeling lighter and younger than they had for years. Therapists have told me that it usually takes this long for people to open up and talk about what's really bothering them. They need the trust and safety of a long-term relationship to bring forth their most troubling material. But for every such person there are others who intuitively recognize the healing potential of meditation and willingly undergo the initiation process of relaxation and catharsis, relaxation and catharsis. In either case, the first and the last steps on the quest are the same: feeling (first bad, then better).

Reaching for the Elixir

The elixir is the substance you drink, eat, or breathe in, that gives you strength to heal and get on with life. It is the missing element you have been craving, the catalyst you need to become whole. Imbibing the elixir is symbolic of restoring your connection with the wholeness of life.

To your body, the elixir may be a vacation, or finding how to use meditation to get the deepest rest you have ever had in your life. It could be finding a way to eat that makes you feel strong and wonderful. To your heart, the elixir may be a deep emotional release that reestablishes the flow of love. To your soul, it might mean being truthful with yourself or having an insight that frees you from guilt or fear.

For some people I have listened to, the elixir is just resting when you need to,

LORIN'S NOTEBOOK

SANDRA AND JANET: REACHING FOR THE ELIXIR

A woman I know, Sandra, described reaching for the elixir of relaxation after teaching second graders all day.

"I looked at the bills on my desk, looked at the TV sitting there, looked at my sofa, and I said to myself, 'You know what? I think I will just take this time for myself.'

"I sat down on the sofa with a book on how to meditate and read about a page before my eyes felt like closing. I just sort of sank into myself. To my surprise, I didn't have a lot of thoughts. I was aware mostly of a buzz of fatigue in my muscles. I uncrossed my legs and put my feet on the floor because it felt like the blood could circulate better that way. As the fatigue slowly percolated out of my muscles, I experienced a rather sweet sensation, an almost musical hum. I sat there breathing with it for the longest time. The sensation of melting spread from my legs and my thighs to my pelvis and lower body. I could feel my butt relax, and my heart and shoulders. My eating only when you want to, feeling good about yourself, or living in harmony with all life. For other people who are addicted to alcohol, cigarettes, or marijuana, to watch them drink and smoke you would think that their substance of choice is an elixir. Maybe it once was. But I think that if you drink water with that kind of reverence, or inhale air as if it were the Magical, Purifying, Enlightening Smoke of All Time, you

body seemed to know what it was doing; I was just enjoying it all.

"Finally, after I had paid attention to my entire body and accepted all the fatigue, the sensations changed to a kind of gushing release, as if I were opening up inside. My mind was almost completely stopped; I was poised there, a little afraid that if I did anything I would spoil the feeling of being permeated by something sweet—the sweetness of life. Sitting in the quietness, I realized that I was happy. 'I have a great, if tiring, life.' I opened my eyes and realized that about 40 minutes had passed. All that evening I felt as if my head was completely clear and I had so much energy. Now I meditate more and more after work, and my evenings are like a fresh start."

To Janet, the elixir of relaxation has replaced the lure of alcohol. She used to drink wine in the evenings in order to relax; she wouldn't really taste the wine, she drank purely for the physical effect. You wouldn't say she was an alcoholic, but she was definitely relying on the wine to provide the relaxation she desperately needed. Now she sips wine but doesn't want to drink too much because she is already having fun. She looks great—fresher, healthier, with good skin tone.

could have just as good a time, maybe better. Try it yourself: Drink a cup of water and pretend it is the elixir of healing.

When you discover how pleasurable meditation can be, the act of meditating can itself feel like the elixir. When I began meditating in the late 1960s, there was a period of 7 years or so when this was a particularly strong experience. I felt drenched in elixir, and as if I had an unlimited amount to give away through lecturing, teaching, and laughing. The sustained joy and openness that I found in meditation led me to forgive everyone, let go of my hurts, and be the person I was meant to be. Then my inner world changed, the wheel revolved, and answering the call meant expressing myself more completely in the outer world and developing different sides of myself than the meditation teacher. I felt called to be a fool, a beginner, an awkward teenager, an explorer with a completely open mind, and not an initiate of the ancient mysteries.

Now meditation attunes me to find the elixir out in the world. My head is often so busy with thoughts that even if I take a walk, I am thinking, thinking, thinking. It's only after a long swim that I am totally cleansed of thought and experience reality as an incandescent, shimmering field of life. Meditation prepares my mind and body so that when I take a walk, when I talk to a friend, when I dance, my being is so tuned in that everyday life is an elixir, a magical intersection of the timeless and the trivial.

This could be you too. Indeed, those who meditate often look like they have been drinking the elixir of immortality.

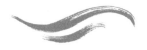

Bringing It Home

The quest is a cycle—we are called, we cross the threshold, we find what we are looking for, and return. The cycle is not complete until we bring the elixir home to our everyday life and restore the wholeness. As you discover the ways in which meditation suits you best, you will develop confidence and self-sufficiency because you are bringing your inner resources up from the depths and making them available in your daily life, where you need them. This is bringing it home, finding the way to bring the revitalization of the elixir into your ordinary world.

It is not enough to experience a few seconds of inner peace during meditation. Everyone has these fleeting moments, after the noise in the head crescendos. Then the next thought comes, or a sound in the outer world reminds you that the clock is ticking and soon it will be time to get a move on. You suddenly remember all the chores to be done, and you are thus on the road home as your being is reorienting to the outer world. Your first challenge is to let the elixir, the sense of repose, permeate the *thought* of the world, the *mental rehearsal* of action. You do this by not resisting thought and by simply enjoying the movie your mind is making of the actions you are to do or have done. By this, you begin to bring peace to your outer life. Then it is time to end the meditation and resume your active outer life. Over time you will find that something is carried over from your meditation into your outer life—a sense of grace in action, greater relaxation, more poise. Other people, your friends and family, will notice that you seem steadier and are more enjoyable to be around. This is bringing the elixir home.

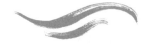

Stress and the Quest

In my book *Breath Taking* I explain why the stress response that we've inherited from our ancestors, and that served their survival, does *not* serve us as well in this day and age. While a lightning-fast physical reaction fueled by a burst of adrenaline is an effective biological strategy for escaping the grasp of a predator, it is not so very useful in dealing with such "threats" as commuting to work, giving a presentation to the group about your project, petitioning for a raise, or asking your sweetheart to marry you. Interestingly, the stress response itself has become one of the biggest killers in countries where modern medicine and sanitation have eliminated most of the dangers to health.

Having to orient, reorient, adapt to new situations, invent new ways of doing things—these are the challenges and the joys of living in the modern world. But the emergency stress response trumps everything; it overrides whatever long-range plans you might have and can throw off the body's sense of timing. A lot of the addictions and bad habits that we adopt are just an attempt to restore our timing (see "Addictions"). Or perhaps you avoid bad habits, but your blood pressure becomes permanently elevated by the stress hormones circulating in your system over a prolonged period of time.

Even slight amounts of stress can make us feel like fighting or running away. The animal in us has only the input from our senses and emotions to go on. If we tell the body that bills, changes at work, and delays in traffic are actual life-threatening dan-

ADDICTIONS

Chronic stress causes chronic problems. If you have experienced stress for a sustained period of time at some point in your life—you fought in a war, you endured a relationship that felt like a war, you were a victim of childhood sexual abuse, you suffered through a terrible divorce or some equally stressful event—you may have developed an adaptation, a repeated behavior. The body can become trapped in a twisted attempt to release itself from chronic tension with what is called an addiction.

Addictions tend to have something good about them, a primitive logic. If the tension was very great, perhaps you developed a habit of drinking alcohol, which is a muscle relaxant. Smoking cigarettes is somewhat relaxing. Overeating, although it is a challenge to the digestive system, can create sleepiness; finally, you rest a bit. Illegal drugs such as marijuana and cocaine are effective painkillers. We can try to lose our pain by rushing a relationship, having compulsive sex, or becoming involved with someone who hurts more than we do.

When such adaptations to chronic tension happen, they are hell to live with and hell to get out of. They can take over and rule your life. All your vitality, your wealth, your life's blood of creativity can be stolen by these behaviors, which started out as an attempt by the body to release stress.

gers, we will have problems—self-generated problems. If this situation continues uncontrolled, it is like we have caged up our inner animal and are torturing it. On top of it all, in the civilized world we are fed a steady diet of stress-inducing propaganda. The media, with their incessant banging away at statistically tiny dangers, may rob years from your life in the way that cigarettes do.

PERSONAL RESPONSES TO STRESS

We all have experienced, at least momentarily, most of these common responses to stress. Some of these reactions may have become bad habits; others we may have faced at some point in life and eventually overcome.

Behavior: compulsive eating or smoking, or else self-starvation and denial of healthy needs; grinding the teeth at night; anxiously scanning the environment when there's no implied threat

Body: sweaty palms, dizziness, ringing in the ears, headache, indigestion, backache, racing heart, fatigue

Emotions: irritability, irrational anger, lack of pleasure, depression, loneliness, powerlessness

Mental functioning: continual worry resulting in difficulty making decisions and thinking clearly; tunnel vision concerning the object of worry, leaving no time for the big picture

Relationships: taking your frustration out on your loved ones, or overloading your relationships with your distress; blaming others; isolating in order to not rage at others; chronic intolerance, distrust, suspicion, and other relationship-killing emotional tones

When our bodies stay in the stress response for long periods of time, our self-repair mechanisms may not function well enough to keep us healthy. The excess wear and tear can eventually lead to stress-related illnesses: backaches, skin disorders, eating disorders, irritable bowel syndrome, insomnia, hypertension, heart attacks, chronic pain, and immune system disorders. Chronic stress can be a factor in bringing on these ailments, and situational stress definitely makes them worse. Stress has also been implicated in a wide range of more minor symptoms (signals) that nonetheless can add up to big problems for you (see "Personal Responses to Stress"). Taken as a whole, the list of stress's negative effects seems overwhelming. Indeed, study after study has shown that about 80 percent of all visits to the doctor involve stress-related illnesses.

Physiologically, meditation is the mirror opposite of the stress response. Blood pressure, muscle tension, breathing rate, heart rate, and metabolic rate all decrease during meditation. It makes sense that the body would have a built-in antidote to the stress response that allows it to repair and recharge its batteries, and here it is.

But meditation does not feel like pure relaxation, because of another function that kicks in. As you relax and come home to yourself, your nervous system does a review of all the times that the emergency stress response was activated. There, sitting in the safety of your chair or on your sofa, you'll find yourself reliving all of the stressful events that have left a residue of bad feeling in your body. This can feel like a subtle form of torture, because the nervous system goes over and over the alarming events until it is satisfied that you have learned all you can from them. If you have made mistakes, you'll see them. If you ever overreacted, you'll see that, and see how you could have done things differently. In short, during meditation you will see movies of tense situations and they will replay until you learn to stay relaxed and breathe easily. If the stress response is called for, then you'll find yourself replaying the situation and applying the exact amount of urgency that is appropriate.

Almost everyone hates this natural occurrence during meditation, and it's a major reason people quit meditating. But such avoidance is based on a misunderstanding of how nature works; that is, how your brain, which is part of nature, operates. The nervous system works constantly during meditation to adapt, evolve itself, learn from experience, and prepare for successful action in the future.

In meditation you deal with things by going right through them. When painful memories come up, just wade on in with all senses alert. Allow the pain to wash through you and be processed by your whole body. If something comes up, just face it, whether it be a demon or an angel. You transcend not by avoiding, but by going directly through. So if you feel stressed, your attention is being called. Go right into the heart of the stress, identify its source, and *feel* what the problem is. Notice what happens in your body and heart and mind.

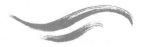

Common Taboos You'll Face on the Quest

In mythic imagery, there are the threshold guardians, fierce entities that make vast amounts of noise while rattling their weapons threateningly when we cross into their turf. They have to be outsmarted or dealt with somehow if you are to proceed on the quest. These guardians present themselves as obstacles, but when you acknowledge their presence and address them directly, a way can be found around or through them.

Whenever you leave familiar physical or emotional territory and enter unknown terrain, there are inner warning signs and signals that say VERBOTEN or NO TRESPASSING or sound off *Ah-O-O-O-gah* or *Ring-ring-ring!* . . . They make you wonder, *Am I really sure I want to cross this line?* To proceed along the healing path, the path to wholeness, you need to say *Yes!* and face the guardians that in meditation take the form of taboos.

If you give it a chance, you may find that your body likes to meditate. But some people have a taboo against self-care. To allow meditation its healing power and to steer clear of self-abuse, you have to confront the taboos that limit intimacy with the self. Because although meditation is healing in a general way, it is more so if you make it responsive to your needs and do not see it as an imposition.

A tip: Never blame yourself when you encounter the following taboos. They are encountered by almost everyone who sets off on the quest for wholeness. When you accept this simple fact and see them for what they are, merely chimeras, their power is transformed into renewing energy you will need on your journey. They may even smile and help you along your way.

The Taboo against Rest

Our jangly culture routinely denies the need for rest. It is a time sickness, an incessant hurrying that is manifested in overloaded schedules and a continual flogging of the self to do more. We are a work-oriented society that worships adrenaline and values being busier than thou as a virtue. Consequently, many people have a sleep debt of dozens of hours.

Meditation brings us face to face with the taboo against rest in several ways. First off, you are sitting there making a science out of doing absolutely nothing. You can read all the Zen koans you want, but when you make your body as idle as it can be, you are sure to run head-on into the taboo against rest. Also, many people choose to meditate at times when others are up and active, either early in the morning or before dinner. It is unusual to be relaxing with your eyes closed at those times—everyone else is watching people being murdered on TV or fuming in traffic. There may be voices, sensations, impulses saying, *What are you doing resting? You should be doing chores!*

Rest is one of the body's most potent resources to accelerate healing. When we are resting, the body can give over its energies to maintenance and repair. We rest every night in order to rejuvenate and recharge for the following day. Sometimes a good night's sleep feels miraculous, because of the way we feel when we go to bed and how fresh we feel when we wake up in the morning. When we are sick, we often have the urge to sleep more, take naps. For their part, doctors love prescribing bed rest.

During meditation we are conscious, fully awake, sometimes superlatively awake, in a heightened state of awareness. Every thought stands out. We are not anesthetized as we would be if we were drinking alcohol or on some other drug. However, the body enters a state of restfulness much deeper than sleep, and it does so very quickly. It is not physically possible, unless you know how to hibernate somehow, to be more at rest than in meditation. You are quite literally doing as little work as possible. That is why the taboo against rest and the taboo against laziness stand sentry side by side.

Something you can do to help your meditation help you is to catch up on your sleep or at least reduce the amount of sleep deprivation you suffer from. Go to bed a little earlier and take naps and rest breaks throughout the day.

THE TABOO AGAINST PLEASURE

Along with a Puritanical work ethic, many people also shoulder a taboo against simple bodily pleasure.

As you relax into meditation, pleasurable sensations will seep deep inside you as your nerves and muscles melt into mush. This often feels like being massaged and drifting in and out of a luxurious sleep. Lying down or sitting when you are tired is one of the sweetest sensations there is, and in meditation you are awake to enjoy it. This world of sensation is as rich as art, music, and wine, which contain infinite nuances of deliciousness. Sometimes your response from somewhere in your brain will be, *No, stop, you can't enjoy this. This can't be right!* You are being seduced by the life-giving energies flowing through your body. Learn to not resist this healing flow. Sensations are not a problem; simply enjoy them. They will change continuously anyway. If you just breathe with the sensations for a minute, they will come to feel normal. Gradually, you will build up your tolerance for bliss.

On a daily basis, indulge in the myriad little pleasures you have available to you. Delight in several such pleasures as part of your preparation for meditation and remind yourself that it is okay to enjoy.

The Taboo against Aliveness

Meditation can feel like a bath in life's rare essence. Even though you are just sitting there, you can feel yourself shimmering, bubbling with impulses. Because you are more open to yourself, you are letting sensations of electricity flow through your body, and this results in intense sensations. As you let go in meditation, your muscles relax, circulation increases, and there are odd tinglings and gushes of life. This feels very taboo, almost too much to handle for most everyone at first.

This fiery side, which we all have, is the perfect balance for the mellowness of meditation, and if you deny it, your vitality will suffer. In order to heal, you may have to risk being more lively than your family, friends, job, or love relationships generally allow. The people who know you may have come to rely on you being low-key, or always kind, or always giving. You should break your own and their taboos.

Whether your injury is emotional or physical, one of the elements you may need to reclaim is your rage to live, which you may have lost as a child or later in illness. In this rage to live there is a demanding quality combined with a healthy zest. Aggression is part of it, being excited about life and reaching out to grab what you want and moving away from what you do not want. To live fully, you have to dare to disturb the universe.

You can feel intensely alive when you are meditating. As a living being, you can demand things of your meditation. You can demand, request, desire, and pray that in a half-hour you will be restored and vivified. Then let go totally and let your body repair itself and prepare to continue the quest.

The Taboo against Spontaneity

Whenever you meditate, be willing to be surprised. The opposite of control is spontaneity, and in meditation it is very useful to have an informal, natural, unfettered attitude toward your inner life. The transition from control, which may be your usual mode of going through life, to release of control, is another threshold crossing with

LORIN'S NOTEBOOK

LAM: SPONTANEOUS HEALING

One of the first people I instructed in transcendental meditation was a physicist from Cambodia named Lam. It was early 1971, and we were sitting there doing his first 10-minute meditation when he started vibrating. His legs jumped around, then his torso got in on the act, then his entire body was vibrating as if he were dancing to Elvis. I was totally unconcerned. I had just come back from a year of meditating and been through lots of shaking myself. The whole feeling in the room was peaceful. I didn't detect anything wrong; there was no sense that he had an illness. So I just sat there and looked at the Pacific Ocean through the window, occasionally glancing over at Lam, who at some point had fallen off his chair and was lying on his side shaking. This went on for about 10 or 15 minutes. I maintained my totally blasé attitude and eventually he stood up, took a breath, and said, "I must have been going through a phase transition. Now I feel very different." Then he sat down and we continued. I acted as if this were the most normal thing in the world, and he had a lively and calm meditation. Over the next year he would occasionally vibrate while meditating, but he never considered it a problem. He owned the vibrating as his own life force freeing itself up.

If you are afraid of being spontaneous, then you probably don't trust yourself and you will not let go as much during meditation. You won't go very deep, and so you won't experience catharsis. This is part of life's wisdom: You only get what you are ready for, so if you are getting it, you are ready.

its scary sensations to endure. As you get used to them, you will find more ability to be spontaneous in your everyday life.

When you close your eyes to meditate, one of the first things that happens is every little thing you have forgotten comes to awareness. You might have several minutes of *Oh no, I left the laundry in the dryer; Uh-oh, I forgot to call Jennie back, she'll be pissed; Whoops, I was going to drop by the mechanic's on the way home to have him listen to that noise the car is making.* There is no telling how long this will go on—it depends on how complex your life is and how good you are at organizing your time. By the way, I recommend that all meditators study time management and have good to-do lists, because it takes a load off your meditation time.

When you release control, your brain's backlog of unprocessed to-do's will take over, and there is no honest way to stop the process. You just have to let it sort itself out. When we are walking around and we remember something we have forgotten to do, it feels like a little hit, a tiny shock going through the body. When we are sitting still in meditation, all relaxed and attentive, the sensation seems more intense. As you get used to it, though, these kinds of thoughts become like rain on the roof—you can hear the constant patter and it's actually quite pleasant.

The process gets worse from here. After your brain gets through your immediate to-dos, it will start to work on long-range desires: *Hey, I promised myself a trip to Europe and I never took it even though I had the money* or *You know, I want a real home* or even *Oh no, I forgot to have kids!*—all those things you have successfully pushed to the back of your mind for years.

You may also have forgotten to give yourself time to feel, in which case you may find yourself crying and not knowing why, or shaking, or getting angry. If you let yourself be taken by your emotions, you don't know where they will take you. The more you let go of control, the more your body will just do what it has to do to balance itself.

What lets you enter a spontaneous mode is trust in your body and your nervous system. The fear of releasing control, just letting the attention wantonly go here and there, feels like an immense taboo. Scandalous!

Because of this, I have noticed that many people make up elaborate rules about what they can and cannot think of during meditation. That's not promoting inner freedom at all. Avoid imposing such arbitrary, restrictive rules upon yourself, because they limit the flow of life considerably and make meditation seem like work rather than recreation.

Then there are some people who are wired so that they will not or cannot allow a new experience to just happen to them. They need to see a map of how it might unfold first, then think about it, decide if they want to go there, get a compass, take a reading, and, if and when they finally set off on adventure, they take it step by step by step by step. A friend of mine is like this. He is extremely perceptive, has done a great deal of self-exploration, and is a very lively guy. But I notice over the years that he never opens up to an aspect of breath, movement, meditation, or sensory awareness unless he decides to and scopes the entire process out in advance. For him, allowing even a relatively minor change in the way he experiences breath is like moving, as in packing up your house and relocating. It's a major operation. To him, a lesser change is like remodeling, maybe knocking down a wall. It causes a mess, and you'd better have a damn good reason for proposing that he make such a change.

I call such people map-firsters or top-downers. They will refuse the call until the call comes bearing maps, logistical details, cost-benefit analysis spreadsheets, brochures, environmental impact reports, insurance policies, and an American Express card. The call then has to wait while the map-firster thinks all this through. When he finally decides to answer the call, he has already done a great deal of the work in advance. He memorized the maps while he was mulling it all over. He has rehearsed what it will be like and given his nervous system permission to accept new levels of perception.

When you perceive a mistrust of spontaneity in yourself or others, be patient. Everyone has his own way and timing for jumping into the dance of life.

THE TABOO AGAINST DESCENT

In dreams and myths, there is the recurring image of descent into the underworld. In meditation, sometimes you may feel as if you are falling. The sensation is similar to

THERAPY

I am a big fan of therapy of all kinds—dance, art, music, massage, group, theater, and talk, to name a few. It's often beneficial to work with a teacher or therapist or coach, not just to learn more about meditation or even yourself, but to enhance your appreciation of anything you love.

what you may have felt when taking a nap or falling asleep, only this time you are falling into meditation. Get used to it.

Sinking down into meditation can feel a bit like depression at times. It is as if there is a vast pool of blackness below you, and you sink into it. This blackness, by the way, is real—much of the universe is vast empty space. Even the matter your body is made up of is 99.99 percent empty space. It's not like reality is solid.

If you have been living in your head, for instance, you should welcome the move into your heart. Or, say you have been using your brain at work all day; 10 minutes into a meditation you may notice that your center of consciousness has slipped down to your belly. This short-term descent gives your brain time off from acting as the center of your being.

There are other descents you'll face in meditation. If you are disabled, you may have the feeling that everything has been taken away. If you are hurt, injured, or ill, you may not be able to do your usual activities. Your motion and pleasure may be se-

LORIN'S NOTEBOOK

ANONYMOUS: REGRETS

Sometimes what you have to heal in meditation is remorse over what you have done wrong and people you have harmed. Guilt that has been eating away at you for years may come up to be suffered with until you do what you can to make amends. Facing these inner demons is excruciating, but only through doing so can we bring our lives into balance again.

I once met a man who told me the following story. "I used to work for a big law firm. My specialty was to destroy the credibility of the people who had been injured and were suing the company my firm represented. I assigned investigators to put together information that would damage the reputation of the injured person, and that would torment them if it were brought up in court. I did this for 18 years. Money was no object. The firm routinely spent hundreds of thousands of dollars on these seek-and-destroy missions, attacking people who had been injured." He paused and then said, "Now I have cancer of the heart." He went on to tell me how he has devoted his life, whatever time he has left, to helping other people as much as he can.

Almost everyone has something to regret, though maybe it doesn't seem this dramatic. When you let down your inner walls, what comes up is your conscience. The small still voice in the back of your mind is a self-balancing force, there to provide course corrections on the path of life. When we run from this self-correcting, the conscience can seem like a demon. When we face it, there is anguish that leads to transformation.

Welcome your demons, and discover how they can become your allies.

verely restricted, either permanently or temporarily. This feels like a small death, a loss, and can result in depression.

If you have been given a difficult diagnosis or prognosis, you may have had a sinking feeling followed by an overwhelming sense of fear. There is a hidden gift in the sinking feeling, because the fear makes us want to run around in panic, which doesn't help.

MEMORY AND HEALING

Has there ever been a time in your life when you felt particularly healthy? Perhaps you have had many such times. What was it like, in both your outer and inner worlds? Take a breath and let the memories come. . . .

Remember the overall feeling of movement in your body, of movement in your life, of going toward your goals. Access the quality of "being with" yourself that you had at the time. Let each of your senses bring you the gift of information about what it feels like, looks like, smells like, and tastes like to be healthy.

If a particular part of your body is giving you trouble, make a special effort to re-create how that area feels when it is healthy. For example, in the times between asthma attacks, how does your breathing feel? If you think about this feeling during the attack, it appears that the body calms down and the symptoms diminish.

Although it may sound too Pollyannaish and more scientific research is sure to come, meditation techniques such as remembered wellness are exactly this simple—and they work.

Depression makes us feel like sitting still and doing nothing, which is at least restful.

There's also descent involved when facing death. The body senses the possibility of death at the end of each exhale. Death comes quickly, in just a few minutes, if we do not breathe in again. We usually flee from this thought because it is too terrifying. But all spiritual traditions say that being aware of one's inevitable death is one of the best preparations for living a full life. It helps you cherish the preciousness of life, however much you have left of it.

Depression is a call in to your depths. Meditation allows you to answer that call safely and consciously so that you can reach to the very foundation of your being and gather the inner resources that are your strengths. In one of the ancient Babylonian myths, Gilgamesh had to dive into a bottomless sea to pick a healing plant. Sometimes you will feel that you are sinking endlessly. As you learn to trust and tolerate these feelings, afterward you will find yourself renewed. If you need help trusting the descent process, I recommend seeking out a member of the clergy, a therapist, or a grief counselor. Let them help you, and then when you are meditating, you will be more skilled in accepting your inner experience. (See "Therapy" on page 46.)

I remember one day in 1972 when my meditations took me into a place of darkness. I was used to inner light and electric sensations, surf and sunshine. This was like being in a cave. Although in the physical world it was light outside, my inner world was dark, silent, vast, other. Slowly, slowly, over months, my body began to make friends with the darkness, to rest in it. Curious, I watched as the cells of my body pulsated in rhythm, contacted the blackness, and then began to absorb nutrition from it. I learned that the darkness is renewing, and a vital ally. There are times on the quest when what we need is a restful immersion in total darkness.

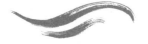

Remembering Wellness

Another important ally to enlist on your healing quest is the power of remembering wellness. This marvelous phrase was coined by the mind-body specialist Dr. Herbert Benson in his mid-1970s classic *The Relaxation Response.* Benson wrote that the *body* has a memory—not just a mental memory but a total cellular recollection of what it is to be well. More significant, the body can actually call on that memory to re-create the state of wellness. If you can remember what you felt in a certain part of your body before it was injured, this will speed your recovery, claims Dr. Benson.

The concept of remembered wellness works on the same principle as the placebo effect. Traditionally, Western medicine has focused on measuring the benefits of an active agent, such as medication, at the expense of the native ability of a patient's belief and expectation. But the presumption that a certain pill, herb, injection, or procedure is going to heal you has been shown to have a measurable effect on many types of maladies. This is called the placebo effect, and it can be evoked by a scientist or doctor in a white coat with an authoritative air giving you a sugar pill and saying, "Take this and you will feel better." Everything from allergies and asthma to back pain, depression, nausea, skin rashes, and a host of other ailments responds positively to a placebo. The placebo effect is especially pronounced if you believe your doctor is giving you a powerful medication.

LORIN'S NOTEBOOK

ROB: WALKING WITH REMEMBERED WELLNESS

Rob Swan is one of the dozens of people I interviewed who are using meditation to cope with illness. Here is one of Rob's favorite meditation techniques.

"When you are ill and lacking in strength and endurance, I find that walking at a natural pace—which will most likely be much slower than one's normal pace when healthy—works as beneficial meditation when all the while you are remembering what is was like to walk before illness set in. The more real the memory, and the more one is able to let that memory sink in to all the cells of the body while walking, the better the results. I've done this, walked slowly—in my mind fully remembering how my body felt when I used to walk home at night after studying at the library when in college—and after my little walk, for a while, I felt like I did when I was young and strong, even as I was weak and tired from the walk. The combination of doing physical movements while remembering how those movements felt when one was healthy is a powerful meditation.

"The more the body can be made to remember what it was like to be healthy, the more the body will be able to access this memory at the cellular level as it tries to repair itself."

Exactly how this works is an immensely intriguing field of research for scientists, who generally credit the placebo effect with creating up to a 32-percent improvement in symptoms. This high level of potency poses a huge hassle for pharmaceutical companies, who have to test every new drug they produce against a placebo. Whatever the effect of the new drug, it has to beat the performance of the placebo. Lots of drugs that are safe and effective fail to make it to market because they just aren't that much better than the placebo—maybe they create a 38-percent improvement, which isn't significant enough to warrant production. Oh well, another hundred million dollars down the drain.

You need to know about the placebo effect for at least two reasons: 1) a 30-percent boost in healing power is nothing to scoff at; and 2) although traditional medicine tries to control for the placebo, almost any medication you take will be more effective if you visualize and feel the drug working. Likewise, the placebo effect of remembering wellness is real. It mobilizes your entire body system and may involve the release of intrinsic healing chemicals such as endorphins, which mediate your perception of pain.

Meditation is often a plunge into pain, because you are deeply relaxed and open to yourself. Whatever is there, you feel. Even if you are perfectly happy and healthy, there is always a lot of wear and tear to be repaired during the restfulness of meditation. Then, after a while, the increased attention results in a reduction of pain. People are often surprised at how well they feel after meditating. You may forget that you are injured or hurt and feel an overall sense of wholeness. This feeling itself has a part in healing—it is a kind of release, a catharsis that helps the body remember wellness. The feeling of extraordingary wellness usually passes after a few hours, but as time goes on you can learn how to stay with it more and more throughout your day.

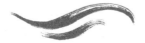

The Sensual Experience of Healing

Each individual has a unique way of experiencing healing. The visceral sense of establishing your connection to wholeness changes every few seconds in the rhythm of your individuality. Here are some general categories that meditators report.

Light. You may experience being flooded by light, bathed in light, massaged by light, merging with light, becoming light. Or you may focus on a particular texture, frequency, or color of light that you cherish.

Sound. You may experience a current of sound that feels like it is tuning you and vibrating away your out-of-tune diseases or pains. You may feel that you are being nourished by resonant sound, and purified by it. You may feel that your soul is singing to you, singing you into wholeness and health. You may merge with sound and experience yourself as vibration, or you may feel it in you and around you, massaging you. You may hear inner urgings calling you home, beckoning you onward and inward.

(continued on page 56)

LORIN'S NOTEBOOK

STEVE: THE JOURNEY FULFILLED

Steve was in his mid-forties and told me he had been meditating for 7 years. His meditation was going well, and he was curious if there was something more he could be doing. I asked him how he started meditating. He said that after working in a pharmacy for a while, he had the opportunity to buy one and run it himself. He built that business up, and then created another, and another. The money was great, but the risks were also; he was under a lot of stress, and he worked overtime to keep everything going.

One day Steve went to the doctor for a routine physical and was told that he was developing high blood pressure and should start taking medication. He said, "Doc, I don't want to start taking that stuff! I know what the side effects are. I see people taking those medications for their entire lives once they go on them. Those are my customers. There must be something else I can do!" The doctor said, "Well . . . you could try this," and he fished around in a filing cabinet and came up with a flyer on how to elicit the relaxation response. "Come back in 4 months and we'll see how you are doing."

Steve had his blood pressure tested a number of times in the next week on different instruments, and the results were about the same, so he knew it wasn't just white-coat hypertension he was experiencing. (This is the phenomenon where being in a doctor's office makes you so nervous that your blood pressure goes up.) So he set his will on making his blood pressure go down without medication. He practiced eliciting the relaxation response—he didn't like the term and instead called it meditating—every day, for 20 minutes in the morning before work and again in the evening. He would just sit in a chair and repeat the word "One" in rhythm with his breathing.

About 4 months later he went back to his doctor and at first didn't say a word about what he had been doing. When the doctor remarked that Steve's blood pressure was now in the normal range, he came clean, and the doctor confirmed that Steve didn't need to take medication if he was meditating.

Steve understood something very important: how to learn from his thoughts. Not having been exposed to any of the rules floating around in meditation circles—almost every meditation book has some of these—he didn't get into a habit of resisting the motions of his mind. If he sat to meditate and ended up spending the entire 20 minutes planning some event, he figured it was time well-spent and he felt much better afterward. He said that in fact, most of the time when he meditates he is thinking, juggling, scheming, and being excited by life. He didn't say this in one sentence. I had to draw it out of him. This was the only point in which he was uncertain of himself. Was it really meditating if he was thinking so much and enjoying it? I said yes, that entrepreneurs have a special dispensation from Buddha to scheme.

Steve connected meditation with his outer life in other ways. When he would find himself thinking of old friends during meditation, he would later call them. When he would fantasize over and over about a particular vacation spot or trip, he would follow through and arrange it. He knew that he had to take vacations; it was part of his program to have a great life and be healthy well into old age.

So when Steve finally asked me, "Well, how am I doing, do you have any suggestions?" I had to reply, "No, Steve, this is the part where the teacher learns from the student."

Touch. You may feel you are being kissed, groomed, or massaged by the Holy Spirit, angelic presences, or by some divine quality of life. You may feel yourself being touched intimately and delicately. There is a laying on of hands, subtle hands of life are rearranging you and healing you with infinite delicacy.

Inner movement. The flow of healing energy through you is alternately cleansing, touching, and nourishing. Or you may become that flow, dissolve into it, merge with it. The motion is the dance of life, the divine dance of the universe, and you are one with it.

The flow of breath. It can feel as if the in-breath levitates you, and the out-breath lets you sink into the ground. All the nuances of receiving are present as we receive the inhalation. All the emotions of releasing are there as we release the exhalation. In this in and out flow of breath are all the issues of merging as the breath becomes part of our blood. Enjoying the flow and pulsation of breath can lead to a sense of dissolution, to becoming one with rhythm so that you are pulse and you are silence. The rhythm can feel musical in all the infinite variations of music: exciting, calming, uplifting, tragic, ecstatic, sorrowful, and infinitely poignant.

Balance. Balance is about orienting yourself to the Earth's gravitational field. It can seem magically delightful, a release into something incredibly precious and easy. Healing, too, can seem like releasing a weight into the gravitational field, letting go, and then feeling lighter. Alternately, healing can feel like sinking down into the ground, surrendering, letting go totally into a blessed relaxation.

In the course of your quest you may experience any one or a combination of sensations that tend to change continuously. That's what this book is: an approach to meditation that helps you be resourceful, so that you will be guided from within to invent the meditation techniques you need. In sessions, I have noted people making up sophisticated and unique therapies on the spot (see "Lam: Spontaneous Healing" on page 42), even though clearly they have never heard of advanced techniques. It's just something their bodies are doing in the resourceful state of meditation.

Your specific way of identifying the presence of healing energy will feel natural to you, intimate. It could feel like accepting a part of yourself you have always hated and feared but now realize is you. Or it could feel like falling in love with life. Like falling in romantic love, whole body healing—the end of the quest for wholeness—is usually not at all what you expect, but you tend to know it when you feel it: relaxing into utter intensity, being carried away, transformed.

2

The Instinct to Heal

Your body—every body—is permeated with the adaptive wisdom of the ages. Whether you think of life as a gift from God or as a vast and miraculous complex of molecules, the trillions of cells that make up *you* are masters of survival. In every moment, without your noticing it, millions of processes are instinctively occurring that guard your health, maintain your inner equilibrium, and give you the energy to go after your goals.

The atoms your body is made out of are virtually immortal. They were formed billions of years ago and will exist until the end of time. The lighter elements in your body, such as hydrogen, were formed in the first moments of the Big Bang. The heavier elements in your body, such as the calcium in your bones and the iron in your blood, were formed by stellar synthesis in spectacular, galaxy-rattling explosions. All the processes we call life and the very cells of your self are the fruit of this cosmic blossoming. Think of that next time you look up at the stars and wonder.

Life is a dance of matter and energy, continually—and instinctively—regenerating and evolving. And, as life naturally adapts itself to different conditions, it transforms not only itself but the face of the world. Nowhere are nature's guiding instincts made more tangible than in this vehicle we call the human body.

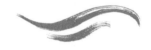

Rebuilding the Body

When you challenge your body, you get fatigued, and then the body rebuilds itself and you come back even stronger. Athletes and bodybuilders take full advantage of this natural instinct to heal in their training and workout programs. Lifting weights, exercising, playing sports—all of these cause microtears in muscle fiber that your body repairs at night and on your rest days. This is the basic principle of strength training. It can take a few days to recover from an intense workout; you may feel sore the next day and really sore two days later.

I remember being surprised when I learned that rest makes you stronger; I'd always assumed it was the workouts that built you up. Physiologists say it's ample rest plus having adequate nutrition feeding the body to provide the raw materials for the repairs. Working out day after day without sufficient downtime can result in over-training injuries, which occur when the body does not have enough time to repair it-self before you stress it again. Coaches and exercise physiologists have done brilliant work in revealing these rebuilding rhythms, and athletes who acknowledge them get better results with fewer disabling injuries.

In daily life we get many kinds of workouts—mental, emotional, and social maybe even more so than physical. We are challenged to cope with demanding environments

In Sync, Naturally

Images from nature often appear during meditation because the body is in league with natural forces. And while we can't see into our bodies to observe the immune system or the digestive tract in action, we can observe many of these same processes at work in nature. For instance, we don't normally hear our hearts beating, but we have a natural affinity for rhythmic sounds. We can't see our blood move through our veins, but we love to look at rivers and streams. We can't see our breath rushing in and out, but there is something enchanting about the ebb and flow of waves on a shore. We don't perceive thoughts as they arise in our brains, but we instinctively feel joy or awe when watching the sun rise.

at home and at work, and we can get worn out on more levels than one. We may ache from fatigue, tension, information overload, or some other factor that affects more than just the body. Mostly the pain goes away by itself; we heal up at nights and on weekends. When symptoms stick around longer or are felt more keenly than usual, the instinct to heal goes into overdrive and triggers a quest for wholeness. This is where meditation comes in. Meditation lets you come back stronger from life's workouts. Among other things, meditation can provide a rest much deeper than sleep that we can access in the midst of our everyday lives to deal with deep distress or disease. The deeper the rest and relaxation, the deeper the healing. When you surrender to sleep, your mind-body system goes on a quest for healing. There, while you are unconscious, the body is free to repair itself thoroughly, and you dream healing dreams. This same process happens during meditation but on a deeper level. Because you are conscious during meditation, you need to learn to consciously cooperate with how nature works, with what healing feels like.

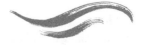

The Power Within

The scientific research on meditation often emphasizes the resting aspect of meditation, because it is measurable and obviously has such a powerful health benefit. Sleep and dreaming are healing, and since meditation is a much deeper kind of rest than sleep, it makes sense that it would be deeply healing. In addition to repairing injured tissue, the mind-body system works on its adaptability and internal stability, preparing itself for action. We experience this every time we sleep and dream, and experience it consciously when we meditate. In the attentive restfulness that is meditation, the brain, nervous system, endocrine system, muscular system, circulatory system, immune system, and digestive system work out their timing and coordination. This is why one simple process of meditation is being prescribed as a treatment for so many different ailments and conditions.

But meditation is not just about the resting instinct; it is something much more exciting. Meditation is the meeting ground for all of your instincts. It is a place where body and soul, all aspects of who you are, come together, at last, to bond and commingle and communicate and work out how to better survive and thrive in this magnificent world. It only makes sense: If nature or God would create beings as complex as humans, then she, he, or it would also provide, as a courtesy, a means to unify the whole mess in harmony and health.

When you are meditating you will notice your experience changing continually and in surprising ways. For a few minutes you may experience your brain sorting through many items on your to-do list, then suddenly you will be in pure repose, a blissful inner quiet. Attention may be called to rest in some part of your body such as your legs or arms or face, and you will enjoy the sensations as the relaxation of meditation massages your muscles into letting go of tension. Then experience will change completely into another need—hunger, loneliness, or tiredness; then after a few minutes you might become excited, sexually aroused, and eager to go live your life with gusto. In this way, meditation is a place where all your instincts meet and greet each other, come to the foreground and then fade into the background, and work out a balance. Understanding this is a central skill in meditation. If you don't accept all this change, all this fluctuation and alternation between instincts, you will tend to struggle against it and have an awful time. Working with the instincts helps give you the inner feedback and skill to meditate safely on your own, with no one to supervise you.

Historically, meditation has been practiced primarily by monks or specialists living in sacred communities or religious orders with close personal supervision. Inner authority was deemphasized, and total, unquestioning obedience to the external authorities was the rule. Meditation was not innate; it happened only by the guru's grace. Most of the classic writing on meditation, West and East, comes from contexts such as this—it is by and for people without day jobs, intimate relationships, bills, kids, or mortgage payments. So of course the whole slant of the classical teaching is toward detachment and against the instincts. As you read, you may find yourself being startled again and again, and thinking, "But wait, this isn't the stereotype of meditation. This isn't the expectation of meditation that I had." Welcome that startle response, for I am using a different language for describing how meditation works, one better suited for people who are practicing on their own, in the midst of their daily lives.

In the modern world, something revolutionary is happening. By far most of the people in the West who are meditating every day do so on their own at home. The meditators of today do not live in Zen centers or yoga ashrams—they live next door. They do not have a guru they see continually—they have to follow their instincts. This is a completely different way of doing things. The path for people who live in the real world is in some ways the opposite of that of a monk—it's toward involvement and appreciation of all the instincts. The instinctive path is about the wisdom of life that you find inside yourself and immediately around you. In truth, the power to heal comes from within.

I know from direct experience that meditation happens naturally. Back in 1968 I

NURTURE THE INSTINCT TO MEDITATE

Meditation feels like time out, time off, a brief vacation from stress or the pain of your ailment. You pay attention almost idly, in the gentlest way possible, to some aspect of the body's self-renewal process, such as breathing, the heart beating, the relationship of your body to infinity, or any of a million other things. In meditation we enjoy whatever the focus is and rest in it. We do so little that the entire *doing* structure of the body is allowed to reset its circuits. The technique is extremely simple, but what can be elusive is finding an approach you love so much that you make time to meditate on a regular basis.

was part of a control group in a brain wave study conducted at the University of California at Irvine. My job was to sit in the dark in a climate-controlled, soundproof room in an overstuffed chair with wires attached to my head for several hours every day for a couple of weeks. I received no instruction or feedback. That's when I learned how to meditate, even if I didn't know it at the time. Later when I heard the word "meditation," I realized that was what I had been doing and started studying the ancient techniques. Over the past 30-some years I have met people everywhere who meditate on their own and are thriving, in spite of having had little or no personal instruction—they learned from within. As I have listened to them talk about their experiences, they have taught me the little tips and tricks that work for them. It is this collective information that I am attempting to put into words here.

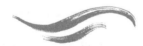

Instincts Lead the Way

Following your instincts helps you answer the call when your body or heart needs healing of some kind. In fact, that's what we call health—when there's a free flow of instincts operating throughout the body. Unfortunately, the workaday world usually conspires against this blissful state, leading us to overwork some instincts while denying others. The resulting imbalance can bring on physical and emotional ailments.

We have many instincts—many different ways of accessing life's mysteries. Probably

LISTEN AND LEARN

When you go to see a healer, doctor, talk therapist, personal trainer, massage therapist, or even a good, wise friend, they usually sense right away what it is you need, and often it relates to balance among the instincts. "You need to play/rest/walk/socialize/have sex more," they might say. Explore this.

there are instincts you do not feel your life can accommodate. Maybe you can't afford to live out your desire to travel, be wild and free, beat people up, or retreat from it all and just stay home. In meditation you can open up a space in your heart to keep your yearnings alive. You may not be able to live them in the outer world, but you can let them flow through your inner world, nourish you, and be integrated with the totality of your being.

A great thing about approaching meditation through the instincts is that all of nature becomes your teacher; animals, plants, the weather, forests, and mountains can give you clues to your inner workings. Remember how in fairy tales and myths the instincts often show up as animals and people who assist you on your quest. They represent the wise motions of life. By understanding what these allies are trying to tell you and where they're leading you, you become a more effective meditator and self-healer.

In the past, meditation was practiced under close personal supervision in closed-door religious communities, and part of the adaptation to life in a religious order was to give up your personal desires. Now, only a small percentage of meditators are working with a teacher, guru, shaman, yogi, or lama. If you are part of the current majority, then your healing authority, power, and spirit must come from within, from following and listening to the instincts.

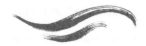

Journeying with the Instinct Allies

When you are meditating, you are face-to-face with the forces that are continually shaping you and forming the texture of your aliveness. The more you get to know these impulses or instincts the more you will be able to accept your healing and rejuvenation. The impulses of life arising in your body want you to be balanced, fulfilled, and healthy, in rhythm with yourself and those around you. The more you trust your instincts and let them operate in the way that is particular to you, the more at home in your body you will feel.

The instincts are allies that help you answer the calls of everyday life. Each has its gift of savvy and energy to give you, or the innate skills of hunting, resting, knowing what to eat, and more. One of the purposes of meditation is to promote a seamless weaving between these instincts and your actions. Your task is to unify them into a working whole to stay healthy or, if suffering, to ignite your natural healing power.

It is most important to let yourself be open and versatile and not restrict your range of responses to the instincts. If you are in need of healing—emotional, mental, or physical—you may have to do things that are out of the ordinary for you. If you let your meditation experience be rich and varied, you are more likely to allow yourself to stretch and do what you need to do to take care of yourself. Besides, the instincts you deny may be exactly the ones you need to turn to for your healing; in fact, this is very likely the case. If you didn't deny them or avoid certain instincts in some way, you would have a natural abundance of that quality as part of your reservoir of healing.

For example, let's go through some of the instincts that you may be neglecting in some way and see how they can affect your quest for wholeness.

Communicating. If you won't talk, you may be keeping secrets from your spouse, friends, doctor, or therapist; you may not be able to unburden your heart and share information vital to your healing. You may not talk to your loved ones and use the time of your hurting to strengthen the bonds between you.

Protecting. If you won't fight for yourself, you may not take the steps necessary to help yourself heal. You may not be able to mobilize your desire to be well, which is often essential on the quest.

Grooming. If you won't care for yourself adequately, your health may suffer. If you won't surrender and let yourself be cared for by others, you may not make time for preventive measures like regular exams.

Resting. If you won't rest enough, you may carry fatigue and stress from one day to the next to the next. Your entire life may be lived under a cloud of tiredness, which affects everything you do and every relationship. If you have injuries of any kind, physical or emotional, your healing may be inhibited.

Nurturing. If you won't make the effort to eat right, really pay attention to what you're eating, then you are hurting your chances for a timely and complete recovery.

For a full, vital life, you want to exercise all of your instincts. Life seeks always to be responsive and adaptable, meaning you can move in any direction you need, and learn whatever you need to in order to thrive. Supple attention is a healthy response to life's callings. Life will be nudging you, so be prepared to feel that nudge, listen to it, move with it. Don't just witness the instincts in a detached way; that will not encourage the flow of vitality through you. While meditating, revel in each instinct as it arises, cherish it, let yourself be moved by it. Use all your senses and the instincts themselves will teach you how to attend to them. Engage them in a playful way and as a matter of course you will discover many fine nuances that no one has ever written about.

Life renews and heals itself by rotating through all these instinctive tones. During meditation, whether you want it or not, your experience will be shaped continually as this rotation occurs. In any given moment, for example, you may be resting very deeply and comfortably in meditation and then a few seconds later the whole tone of your experience changes toward alertness, as if you were hunting or standing guard. Learn to recognize and cooperate with each of these instinctive tones.

The Instinct to Explore

All animals explore their environments, but apparently human beings were at the front of the line when God handed out the instinct to inquire, wonder, and explore. As an individual, you may or may not have activated your own talent for exploration. It could be that your ancestors and the family you were born into had already mapped the great things in life, and all you had to do was take advantage of it. Maybe you have friends who have scoped out the world and told you about it.

If your energy has been stagnating because you don't explore, then make sure to add this quality to the mix of attention you bring to meditation. In meditation, it is up to you to explore and find the sensory pathways that delight you and lead you to healing.

Wonderful Breath

Take a breath now in the spirit of wonder. Explore. Sniff around and see what elixir you can find in your breath right now. Explore the full range of all your senses as they inform you of the breath flowing in. If you are truly awake, each breath will have a fresh quality, like a different batch of wine or crop of fruit than the one before.

There is a reflex that all animals have—the "what's up?" response. You lift your head and look around, all your senses open. This is a kind of exploring where you scan the outer environment for anything new, possibly a threat. When you go inside, explore for the possibility of pleasure, and be awake to whatever is calling you.

When you are in meditation, think the word *explore* a few times. Repeat it in your inner thoughts, or say it quietly using your vocal chords. Think of all the qualities of exploration, then bring your attention to your breath and associate those qualities with your breathing. Say, *I am on an adventure, seeing new lands. I am mapping new pathways within myself. I am open to new experiences and I trust my navigational skills to show me the way.*

The Homing Instinct

When you are moving in your outer world, the homing instinct manifests itself in the craving to return home and your ability to find your way home. This implies that you have a map of the world that includes the distance and routes between destinations. You have some sort of internal compass to determine directions, and you have an internal clock or timing sense telling you when to return home. Separate from homing, but related, is the nesting instinct, concerning the desire to have a home and to make yourself safe and snug there. Whenever the desire arises in you to go home, it is part of a whole set of intelligent orienting responses built into your body that have to do with navigating, traveling, and then taking care of your needs once you arrive. We experience physical and emotional relief when the homing instinct is satisfied. What, for you, are the qualities of being at home? Perhaps when you are at home you move at your own pace and in your own rhythm. You let down your guard and you don't have to act fancy for anybody.

This same sense of relief applies to the inner world if you let meditation be a place where you can feel at home. As you get used to the way your body feels when you med-

HOMEWARD BOUND

Consider the sensations and impulses that arise in your body in the following circumstances: You are traveling, and after a few minutes, hours, days, weeks, or months, you have the longing to be home. As you travel toward home, at a certain point you begin to feel that you're almost there. Then you come to where you can see home: see the neighborhood, your driveway, your house. You approach the door. Walking in the door, you greet your waiting family, friends, dogs, cat. Or maybe there is no one there. You wash up, ex-crete—the relief. Sitting down for a bit, you rest, nest. Settled in and settled down, maybe you make something to eat; drawing in nourishment first by smell and then by taste. There's socializing, sharing news, storytelling, or watching TV and following the story of the electrons on the screen. (What is most interesting in a story is the way the main character is presented with a challenge and then gears up to meet it.) Bonding. Getting intimate with your beloved. Touching. Grooming. Communing. Playing with each other. Tender-ness. Massaging each other. Lovemaking. In moving through life, we travel seamlessly from one instinct to the next, hardly noticing the transitions.

itate, your homing instincts will kick in. You will find the way to your home inside, and make yourself at home. You can learn to be truly at home with yourself in meditation. How can you cultivate this? By being unhurried in everything concerning meditation, including reading this book, and by doing things at your own speed. Always grant yourself a sense of leisure. Be informal, and give yourself freedom to make mistakes.

Physically, make yourself comfortable. Make the chair, sofa, or bed you are sitting on a place of sanctuary. Let your posture be relaxed. Shift around to feel out the position you really want to be in. Emotionally, make yourself comfortable by framing what meditation is in a way that appeals to you. *I am going to just be with myself for a while.*

Since *home* is such a harmonious word and it has *om* in it, chant the word *home* or *homing* softly for 3 minutes. Then let the outer sound fade away and listen to the word in your mind. I think *home* is a better mantra than *om*. When you find yourself being at home in meditation, linger on your way back into the world. Open your eyes and savor the moment and let that which is within spread around you. Stay there for a couple of moments before moving, speaking, or getting back to the flow of the day.

THE INSTINCT TO REST

Life is a rhythm of activity and rest, and we dance through this rhythm all day and all night. Human beings need an amazing amount of sleep to function at their best, usually 7 to 8½ hours per day—almost a third of the day! And there are many

LET THE SUN SHINE IN

In surfing, one thing you do is paddle out, stay out as long as you can, then come in and lie on the beach, soaking up the warm rays of the sun. If you have ever been in cold water for an hour or longer, you know how ecstatic it is to finally flop down on hot sand and surrender.

As a young man, I certainly was not a relaxed person; I was very intense and tense. Perhaps experiencing the dynamic cycles of cold/hot and rest/activation (see page 169) over the course of a lifetime has trained me in how to let go.

times when we need to take a short rest break to renew and refresh ourselves.

The impulse to rest is nature's way of telling us to stop for a moment to tune up our physical, mental, and emotional machinery. We have been designed so that it's quietly ecstatic to sit down and rest when we are tired.

In meditation, you can ride these cycles of activation and rest. They always occur together, and even if you are extremely at peace in meditation there will be little waves of minute activity fading into rest, over and over.

There seems to be a point in every meditation when the brain finally gets done reviewing action and then, without warning, you are invited in to experience the deepest rest you have ever known in your life. You may feel like you are falling asleep, and indeed you may find yourself nodding off. You may notice nothing at all, no thoughts, nothing—you are a pure ball of peace sitting there.

If you meditate at the same time every day, your body will start to call for it around that time. One thing many meditators do when they come home in the evening is to shower, lie down and nap for 10 minutes, and then meditate.

You may find after a while of meditating that your experience of napping changes. Because you have been practicing sensory awareness, when you lie down to nap you may fall into a delicious, slightly awake sense of drifting. Learn to revel in the sensations of restfulness, near napping, and falling into and out of brief meditative naps.

As a focus for meditation, find the most restful things and the most restful ways of being with them. Jesus said, "Come unto me, ye that labor and are heavily burdened, and I will give you rest."

I can rest in myself. I don't have to be on duty in any way. I am safe to rest here. I take refuge in God, in nature, in the Buddha, and rest there.

THE GROOMING INSTINCT

The grooming instinct shows up in bathing and cleansing, combing the hair, attention to clothes, and touch of all kinds that we give ourselves and others. Getting a massage or a facial is grooming, as is having your hair done. Even being examined by a doctor or dentist is grooming behavior. Apes carefully groom one another's fur, and zebras gently use their teeth to remove ticks from one another's backs. Grooming each other is one of the great joys of being in a relationship.

Many phases of meditation feel like grooming, as though in your inner world you are being massaged and bathed by life, breath, and currents of energy. You feel like you are being put all back together again. In the yoga traditions there are extremely elaborate charts of the energy currents in the human body, with details of how they are straightened out and made to flow properly by meditation. The yoga asanas are a sublime way of grooming the physical body and the subtle energy currents that flow through every nerve and muscle. Meditation feels like a total head-to-toe massage every day, and I think this is part of the healthy glow that meditators so often have, like they are drinking from the Fountain of Youth.

To prepare for meditation, you can enact such grooming rituals as stretching, showering, rubbing lotion all over your body, or wearing special clothes. Let tender appreciation of your body be your guide. Meditation will alert you, if you let it, to incredibly subtle nuances of what it is to be groomed from the inside. As you explore how you like to be touched, where and when, you will also learn about how other people like to be touched.

I bathe in the breath of life, I am washed with silence. Let God massage peace into every cell of my body.

THE INSTINCT TO HUNT

Everyone has a favorite form of hunting, whether it be hunting for a video to watch, for information on the Internet, for just the right dress or pair of shoes or earrings to wear, or for the ideal restaurant to celebrate at. You might be hunting for a mate or a job or a house or a bargain. Your senses open wide when you're hunting, and you become alert for tiny clues.

There are many discrete aspects to hunting that make it so interesting. Hunting involves desire—cherishing an image of what you seek. Then you start to follow trails, sniff, listen, look, and pause frequently as you attune yourself to your environment and seek to blend with it. Ancient hunters would draw animals on cave walls and dance in trances to ritually tune themselves to their prey and its methods of moving through nature. In this way they would enter the sacred world with immense respect for the vast powers of nature.

To find what you need in meditation on any particular day, you may need to hunt inside yourself. You may need to wait, as poised as a hunter by a game trail, for the signal that calls you into your inner sanctuary. The ability to wait, senses alert, without impatience yet completely ready for action is invaluable no matter what you do and can make a huge difference in your life. So much of your success in both your inner and outer worlds depends on your ability to listen, actively listen, rather than just waiting for a chance to butt in.

Before you meditate, it is okay to have a goal you are seeking. There can be one thing or many things that you passionately desire. You can even dedicate the meditation to attuning yourself to the fulfillment of that desire. Like the ancient hunters, imagine yourself already at one with what you seek, at one with it in the spirit world.

I am free to hunt for the technique I need today. I can tune myself to my desires so that I have more ability to fulfill them appropriately in the world.

THE INSTINCT TO GATHER

There is a primordial impulse to gather nature in our arms—berries, flowers, grasses, herbs, nuts, fruit—and bring it back to the nest. In the modern world, gathering often takes the form of shopping. Hoarding is an aspect of gathering—deliberately stocking up on anything you think might be handy in case of an emergency.

In contrast to hunting, foraging can be a very low-key activity, even thoughtful. You stroll along looking for certain plants. Blueberries don't run away or fight back ac-

THE MORE THE MERRIER

Teachers of particular schools of meditation tend to get stuck using a limited range of instinctive tones—surrender, ego-dissolution, nurturing, rest, or protection. Every school has its own two or three instincts it adopts, and it tends to ignore or scorn the rest.

The psychologist Abraham Maslow said, "If the only tool you have is a hammer, every problem begins to look like a nail." In meditation, if the only instinct you know is to protect yourself, then every problem will look like a life-or-death threat. To gain a clear picture of your emotional, mental, and physical states and to maintain whole body happiness and health, you need to be in touch with all of your instincts—every one.

tively. If there is an abundance of food in nature, you wind up thinking about who back at the camp will like this kind of berry, that variety of nut, who would want leafy vegetables, and what sort of dishes to make with the bounty. It is a slow and steady process, and you have to plan for how much you can carry. Although hunting parties could be gone for days, gathering parties mostly operated within a half day's walk of camp.

Explore gathering in the outer world; go shopping for food in an extremely relaxed, sensuous way, letting the vibrations in your hands and your sense of smell tell you which are the best vegetables and meats to bring home for your family.

Much of meditation is actually gathering, gleaning from the breath the energies, inspiration, calmness, and vital substance you need to live each day. The Chinese traditions of tai chi and chi gung have developed the skill of gathering energies of breath to a high degree, and it is impossible to praise the genius of tai chi too highly. The fundamental insights of tai chi are accessible to anyone. Sit or stand somewhere, at home or in nature, and hold your arms out in front of you, palms turned inward toward your chest or throat. As you breathe in, gently move your hands in toward your torso. As you breathe out, move your hands away from your torso. Continue this way for 10 minutes and notice what you experience. A few minutes of this is a good way to begin and end every meditation.

As you become attuned to the gathering instinct, you will find certain places in meditation of so much energy that you can pause there and gather it into your body, as much as you can hold. In these moments, act as if you have all the time in the world.

I select from life's cornucopia the materials I need for my growth and healing. I take what I need from life's huge fields and leave the rest for others. There is an abundance of what I need, and plenty to share.

THE INSTINCT TO NURTURE

After hunting or gathering, you take into your body the substances that nourish and revitalize you and you give yourself time to digest. In the outer world, there is the joy of eating and drinking. When you savor your food with gusto, it feeds you on many levels at once. All the gustation—the active sensual pleasures of smelling, tasting, chewing, and swallowing—are a great aid to digestion. One thing I notice in my fellow Americans is that they so rarely take the time to enjoy their food. If you eat mindlessly, you miss half the fun and some of the nutrition, and in fact many illnesses are related to improper digestion. You can sit down to eat the best food in the world, but if you don't give your body time to digest it, you might as well be eating junk food.

In the inner world, there are many energies to feed on and imbibe, many elixirs to taste. Self-nurturing is about receiving and letting the incoming energies be transmuted into a form that is perfect for you. Certain sounds, colors, and ways of breathing may feel nurturing. Each part of your body may crave to be nurtured in a different way. The more you activate this instinct, the more it will guide you to the energies you need to be whole and strong.

There is a satisfaction in the outer world when you have eaten something you really crave and it really hits the spot. There is a similar satisfaction in the inner world when you give yourself permission to feed on the qualities you crave. And as with the outer world, any enjoyable experience deserves time to be digested. One huge mistake I see people exploring yoga and meditation making again and again is not giving themselves time to digest. They jump up and race off with a gnawing feeling of being unfulfilled.

You can help yourself immensely by simply developing the habit of meditating for a minute before or during each meal. Give yourself over to totally savoring the food.

I can receive exactly what I need. I can breathe easily and enjoy the time as my body digests. I do not have to race off, not just yet.

THE INSTINCT TO EXCRETE

Fortunately, the body knows how to get rid of what it no longer needs. Whatever element is overabundant or in a form the body cannot use is excreted. When we breathe out, the excess carbon dioxide is carried away. When we urinate or move our bowels, the old materials are carried away.

Meditation has the purifying, cleansing, and utterly relaxing quality of a good bowel movement. There is the feeling of releasing and letting go. This never occurred to me until one day when I found myself talking to a rather hard-core Alcoholics Anonymous men's group. The men were all former bikers and they sat there smoking and listening to me with great sincerity, but they weren't getting it. They were totally dedicated to the 12 steps, loved the program, but my words on meditation weren't resonating. We did some brief meditation exercises, and I could tell that talk of sunshine and flowers didn't mean much to them. I had a brief impression that what they see when they close their eyes are wild scenes from the past, but what they couldn't see was how letting such images flow through them could have anything to do with spirituality.

Minutes were going by. If you've ever had to speak in public and you lost your audience, you know what I mean. Finally I looked at one man who had a beautiful, ravaged, craggy face, and I followed a hunch and said, "In meditation, what you are doing is letting your brain take a dump." Immediately they got it. They all laughed and relaxed. "You just sit there and answer nature's call. Your brain, your emotional body, it just takes a dump, lets go of the old stuff, and you'll feel a lot lighter afterward. Check it out."

Then we did a meditation and they were totally comfortable. They all needed to

GOING TOO FAR

Large sections of the alternative health movement are fanatically obsessed with colonics and purification of the bowels. This is an instinct taken to the extreme, and it can be dangerous as well as a waste of time. I think this urge may develop out of undiagnosed eating disorders arising from a desire to purge intolerable emotions and experiences.

let go of tension, they were becoming new men, and the old stuff, the dead cells from their previous drunken lives, could be flushed away.

That was the chunk of information they were missing. Although I had never thought of it quite that way before, the idea is all over pranayama, the breath-control exercises of yoga. Lots of yoga breathing is like having a high colonic with pure life energy.

In meditation, you will find yourself flowing through rhythms of feeding, resting, and excreting. Sometimes it may feel like things dropping from your body: *That took a load off my chest.*

If you feel clogged up, emotionally constipated, you can take your time to enjoy the outbreath, which is respiratory excreting. You breathe out every 5 seconds or so—let the outbreath teach you about letting go on all levels, physical, emotional, and mental.

With this outbreath I release all the old air, the old feelings, the old thoughts. I let myself be emptied that I may be filled again.

THE INSTINCT TO PLAY

Play is how all higher mammals practice the actions they need for survival. The young play; they hunt and stalk and leap and frolic and even chew on one another at times. Adults engage in conversations that can have a playful feel. There are many interesting tones of play, innumerable forms of make-believe. Play can be intensely competitive, as in sports, or the most lighthearted thing in the world. I think play is sacred because of the remarkable absorption so many people experience in playing and in watching

PLAY WITH YOUR HEALTH

Many of the most profound healing techniques, including remembered wellness, are really forms of play. "Okay, pretend that your knee/throat/hip/shoulder is perfectly healthy and imagine how it would operate. Now rehearse that motion." If you attach electromyographic detectors to the injured part, you can see the nerves rehearsing normal motion.

Many meditators love variations on this theme: "Go into your imagination to your own special island, and once there go to the temple of your innermost heart. On the altar is a note that holds the key to your healing. What does it say?" The entire Yoga Sutras can be seen as play: "Meditate on the space permeating your body and become as light as cotton. Meditate on strength and become as strong as an elephant. Meditate on the Pole Star and gain knowledge of the motion of the stars."

play. Not everyone is a world-class athlete, but much of the population can be hypnotized by watching someone run, carrying a ball, from one spot to another. In play we exercise our grace, skill, faith, dedication, teamwork, and a whole litany of other attributes that reflect the best in human beings.

Play can be purely internal and imaginary. We can lie down and mentally rehearse an action, such as shooting hoops at the gym, and improve measurably. This may be part of what the brain is doing while we dream at night—running things by, playing around to find the best connections between actions, instincts, and impulses.

Play is the most neglected instinct in meditation. So many people try to keep a straight face and make the tone monotonically heavy. This is to their deficit, because play loosens up all the mechanisms and organs of perception and action. Play is not trivial—it is essential. You can play in any instinctive tone, and play often offers a magic ingredient that helps things work out.

Make sure to give yourself room to play in meditation. It's all your sandbox. You'll discover things goofing around that you can learn no other way. Play with postures, play with breath, play with sound. Play with dancing before you meditate. Wiggle when you're done.

The spiritual masters I have met tend to be incredibly funny. It's as if it takes their supernatural calmness to keep them from cracking up. I laughed for about a year after learning to meditate, after I got a sense of the cosmic nature of things. Everyone, including me, was running around pretending that this little world is all there is when really the soul is at play in this world. It was the funniest thing I had ever perceived. Many people I know have had the same experience, and some are still laughing.

The universe and all of space and time are my playground. I can pretend to my heart's content. I can become completely absorbed in my play, and then, when it is time, I will return to the mundane.

THE INSTINCT TO PROTECT

The protective instinct can be a beautiful thing, as when parents or teachers watch over children in a park so they can play and be themselves; even children can play more freely when they have the sense that they are safe to do so. But the modern world, and particularly our modern media, is prone to take advantage of the protective instinct. Even though people are actually safer than ever before, according to the statistics, most will tell you that they don't feel safe. Many Americans will angrily deny being safe, and they will list all sorts of dangerous things they have heard about on the news. This is because any news organization that reported the straight truth would go out of business. Imagine this top story: "Ninety-nine percent of humanity got up this morning and went to work as usual. . . ." Yawn. Change the channel. Communications theorist Marshall McLuhan pointed out that one of the purposes of the news is to aggravate your instincts, make you afraid, and then sell you things—the products being advertised seem like ways to protect yourself.

SAFETY FIRST

The feeling that you can protect yourself if needed encourages deeper meditation. Do little things to protect your meditation space and time. Train people to not interrupt you, and create a sense of safety for yourself. Many prayers and psalms have a protective quality and evoke powerful feelings of being watched over and wrapped in a safe boundary.

The martial arts have many energy exercises and meditations to develop the sense of protection and strengthen the ability to protect oneself and others. There is a saying in several martial arts, namely karate and aikido, "Relaxation is the strongest state." This is from people who can break bricks or dare people to try to push them over, so heed their words.

During meditation, your nervous system will process all the information it has about the dangers in your environment. You may notice, if you watch the news a lot, that too much of your time is spent damping down the false alarms created by the ghost stories the media is forced to tell. Meditation will remodulate your sensory nervous system so that you are more attuned to the real dangers, slight or great, in your actual environment. You have to be extremely relaxed to have really good intuition; otherwise, the noise and false feelings of emergency will be blaring in your system, overwhelming the quiet signals that are the real clues to what is going on.

There is nothing that adds noise to your head like boundary invasions. When people inappropriately intrude on you, it's infuriating. The boundary invasion can be as simple as a telemarketer calling just as you sit down to dinner, or it can be as offensive as being pulled over because of the color of your skin. In such cases, if you don't respond immediately and push the offender away or snarl at him, that energy

GUT RESPONSE

Inappropriate touching, sexual advances, and even suggestive comments can be infuriating when you are at work, to a degree that's way out of proportion with their seemingly slight nature. That's because you feel trapped and cannot mobilize your full resources to defend yourself. If you could slap the wise guy silly in front of everyone—now that would be satisfying, especially if done within a minute of the offense.

can become stuck in your body. Then when you meditate, that's what you feel—the suppressed snarl. Instead, let your aggression flow so it can serve you.

A woman in her late forties said, "I don't like to hurt people's feelings. I treat other people as I want to be treated. But some people don't get it. They take advantage. I always feel better after meditation, but my mind is very noisy; I have a lot to wade through. One day I noticed how angry my thoughts were and I realized how I let people walk all over me sometimes. I realized I wanted to say, 'Back off,' to this woman at work, but I have never said that to anyone. I felt horror at the idea of actually saying that."

If not addressed, boundary invasions can trigger compulsive behavior: drinking, smoking, overeating, sexual acting out, as well as raging and consequent depression. Meditation can help heal addictions and the trauma of sexual abuse by providing a safe haven to feel. This is why meditation is a part of many 12-step programs. Meditation is the act of touching with infinite gentleness those places inside you that are calling out, screaming to be touched and healed, and as you tend to yourself in this way, the energy behind the compulsions is drained away.

The instinct to protect yourself includes being on guard and being alert at the very instant you are being invaded, whether it's by a salesperson or a pushy worker at the office. Dealing directly with boundary invasions throughout the day will reduce the number of noisy thoughts you have in your head during meditation. Pay attention to these moments and learn all you can from them, for the problem will always be with

THE BEAUTY OF BOUNDARIES

Crossing boundaries isn't always a negative experience; sometimes it can have an exquisite feel to it. What is sweeter than loving someone and wanting them to reach out and touch you more, grab you harder, kiss you passionately? You can really feel your boundaries being magnetized when you are with someone you love and you are sitting together, not touching, and the urge to touch keeps building and building.

you. Learn to make yourself safe, by skilled awareness, in your life and through meditation.

I can move in any direction I need to in order to protect myself and my loved ones. May this meditation make me alert and peaceful so that I can be a source of strength and comfort, allowing others to thrive.

THE HERDING INSTINCT

All people want to belong to something larger than themselves, some tribe, group, or clan. Human beings are wired to be social. Even monks sitting alone on the hillside are members of their spiritual order and are cared for on inner levels by the ancient ones.

Biologically, a human being is a collection of internal organs, each of which is alive and has its own place and function in the body. We are a collection also of trillions of single cells, each of which is a life. Psychologically, a human being is an assembly of many different beings. We see them in our dreams—everyone in a dream is us: We are the writer, producer, and actors. We contain the seeds of all human possibilities.

Meditation is basking in community on all these levels. Much of your time in meditation will be spent sorting through your relationships: how they change, who is dominant, who is zooming who. Another level of sorting you will find your body and mind doing concerns the dominance hierarchies among your chakras, the Sanskrit term for your endocrine system and major organs. Is your head or your heart dominant? What is the place of your genitals in the scheme of things, or your power center? Which chakra gets to express freely, and which has to be the servant of the others? Which has too much energy or too little?

When you meditate, your energy will be called here and there in your body. Part of what is being worked out is the relationship of the parts to the whole, the chakras to the body. In one moment, the energy and love of the entire body is needed to get through to some scared, terrorized, traumatized part of yourself, perhaps your belly or heart. In another moment, the challenge is to get your genitals, with their magnificent, electric sexual energy, to work in coordination with your heart, as informed by your head.

As you are meditating, all this will happen spontaneously in your being, as fast or faster than you can perceive. This process can seem like noise or distraction, but it is not. It is actually your herding instinct sorting through all the various relationships and energies so they can find where they belong in the whole.

I am part of the universal choir. I am one with all those I love. Here in the silence of meditation I cherish my connection to others.

THE INSTINCT TO COMMUNICATE

In the outer world, communication is everywhere at all times. Animals call out to each other. The whales in the ocean sing songs that carry for thousands of miles. Human beings have so much communication going that your body is right now being penetrated by thousands of frequencies carrying our signals. You could put a radio crystal in a tooth and pick up hundreds of radio stations. You could put a phone scanner near your body and pick up thousands of calls. I live on a bike trail near Los Angeles airport, and people rollerblade, bicycle, scooter, walk, and run by while talking on their cell phones. I think that there is an instinct to just gossip. Some birds, by the way, imitate the sounds they hear, and in parts of the world they are imitating the musical ring of cell phones.

When you meditate, you are walking in on a conversation that has been under way for some time. The different parts of your brain are talking to one another; your different organs and glands are talking to one another; the thymus gland is talking to the adrenals, and the gonads are talking to the heart. It's a buzz of conversation. The tone can feel like chatter, gossip, deep communion, or subtle vibrations. Even silence, a resonant silence, is a form of communication.

Contrary to popular opinion, your job is not to get them all to shut up. As the host of this party, your job is to join in while at the same time making sure that everyone has food and drink and another to talk to. Your job is to create a welcoming, warm atmosphere so that the gossip continues. At the very least you should say, "Talk among yourselves," and go about your business of focusing on breath or whatever. Much of the noise you hear or feel is your various energy centers, your chakras, the different brains, catching up on the day.

Encourage communication of every kind, on every level, throughout your being. Encourage intercourse, exchange.

If while meditating you feel a too-much sensation in an area of your body, know that this is often related to the need to express yourself. Expression means that the unit you know as yourself releases her energy into her chosen group by "saying" what's on her mind—or dancing it, singing it, or doing it.

I welcome the communication among all my parts. I celebrate the free flow of information within my being.

THE INSTINCT TO LOVE

When we are in relationship to anything, there is the possibility of love. The other entity could be a dog, a flower, the sun, the ocean, a child, a marriage partner, anything. In love we are led to cherish the other, even above our own lives. We dedicate ourselves to their well-being.

The instinct to love inspires us to appreciate people and to want to bond with them. We want to form a relationship with what we love, and this is as true in the inner world as in the outer. In a love relationship, you can sit together in the silence, enjoying each other's company, or you can talk or do things. The love flavors everything.

When you are dealing with your inner world, there is no rule that you have to be in opposition with all you find there. Beware of teachings that suggest that you de-

MEDITATION AS LOVE

Meditation is always in the service of love, even if love is manifested differently in every person. Love is a state of receiving from the world and giving back to it with all your heart. Love can be about making babies and caring for them—and all the actions prior and subsequent to that, and love can manifest itself as creativity in any realm. Love shows itself in your work, in the urge to protect the people you care for, in science, and in art.

Love has much to do with accepting things as they are, people as they are, and yourself as you are. Meditation facilitates that all-important shift from trying to change things and people and yourself to fit an ideal—which is the road to hell—to making a contribution, any contribution, and doing what you can to create a better atmosphere for everyone, including yourself, to thrive in. This quality of acceptance may be one of the most underrated gifts of meditation.

People who love have a natural gathering instinct guiding their meditation. They seek out and absorb much more energy than they need so that they have plenty to share with the people around them. This is one of the great, relational joys of meditation—having so much to give that you are overflowing with love.

clare war on parts of yourself. That's what led some of the ancient meditators to leave everyone and go sit on a mountain. These teachings (still in print today) reflect their self-hatred disguised as spirituality.

If you have conflicts within yourself, issues to be worked out between what you want now, as a human being, and what some other part of you wants, the tone of love and respect can still permeate the interaction.

Meditation is the practice of love. You do this by paying attention in a loving way to whatever comes up from moment to moment. All the tones of love will be called forth: compassion, passion, tenderness, eros.

Sometimes the proper response to an inner feeling is to love it erotically. This isn't something you have to decide—you'll just be meditating along and suddenly your body is gushing with sexual electricity. What is sex? It is the desire to have love be consummated, a full bodily embrace with nothing held back. Sometimes that is what it takes to get through to relaxation. Sometimes sexual energy is the only thing that will make the connection between the soul and the world.

Arrange for meditation to feel like being in the presence of that which you love. One day, make lists or arrange photographs or just make a series of images in your mind of everything you have ever experienced that inspired you to feel unconditional love, whether it be a dog, a baby, a garden, a poem, a symphony, whatever. Drench yourself in the feeling of unconditional love and breathe with it, memorize it, feed on it, let it become part of you and the ruling passion of your meditation. Associate that feeling with a technique of meditation—a way of breathing, a word, a name of God, so that you can return again and again to bathe in the ocean of love. Let love carry you deeply into meditation.

What love will alert you to are the nuances and combinations of elements, senses, and instinctive tones that are the magic key to your individuality. To love completely, you need to both give and receive love. You may be good at one or the other. Do you give but feel that you don't receive enough in return? Meditating with the love impulse will teach you to be balanced in giving and receiving. If we like to give but don't let others give to us, their hearts may ache with their unfulfilled need to be giving.

You need to find your unconditional love because that is what is required in order to enter the body and stay there in the face of the world's terrors. This requires all the love you have.

I bathe in the ocean of love. I drink it in. My pores are filled with love, and my heart beats and pulses in the fluid of love.

THE GOD INSTINCT

The God instinct is an innate urge to relate to the vast infinity of life in some way. This is beyond curiosity and wonder—it is almost a tropism, a turning toward the ultimate source of nourishment.

The God instinct often calls us without our knowing. We may ache and not know why, or we may think it's alcohol, or drugs, or money we want when what is truly calling us is the need to connect to a higher power. In addition to the herding instinct, which directs our desire to connect with others, we also crave a relationship with something greater than ourselves. This is not just an emotion, for the reality is that we live in a universe that is inconceivably large, and yet we are inseparably a part of it. All of the other instincts lead to the God instinct, if you follow them to their source. Eating, drinking, lovemaking, communing, homing—all have divine aspects, transcendental, that lead you beyond yourself into infinity.

Religions and spiritual traditions are ways of celebrating and ritualizing our connection with this wholeness of life. Your religion of birth, whatever it is, contains utterly ravishing thoughts you can use as your focus in meditation. The names of God are one thing when you say them out loud, another thing entirely when you listen to one of them being whispered in your heart. There is a sonic quality to the inward resonance of *Allah*, *Elohim*, or *Ishwara* that is so exquisite, you feel as if you can listen forever.

If you are religious, then let meditation be in the service of your relationship with that larger world. Cultivate in particular the qualities of surrender, gratitude, awe, and communion as they are pointed to in your tradition. If you are not religious, think of the higher power in your own way, and breathe.

Science tells us mind-boggling stories about our oneness with all life, even distant stars: The air we are breathing at this very moment was born in the heart of mature suns and then scattered into space as they died.

Lately, the most awe-inspiring objects of contemplation I know of are the Hubble photographs of deep space. The universe is so ravishingly beautiful. Astounding images are available for free downloads or online viewing at many Web sites.

I am part of the vast infinity of life. I am immersed in the infinity of the universe. I accept this breath as a gift from God.

FORGING AN EASY ALLIANCE

Much of your success in every area of your life is related to your ability to listen—to listen to what people want, including what *you* want. One important aspect of listening is to be completely attuned to what is being said and also what is not being said. Listen to the feeling and the yearning behind the words, and don't just wait until you can interrupt. Really listen.

Listen to the instincts. The instincts are movements your body knows how to make. Even when you are sitting absolutely still in meditation they will be resonating in you like the echoes of a vast symphony or the hum of the Big Bang vibrating everywhere in the cosmos. You no more need to silence the music of the instincts than you need to tell the universe to stop reverberating so you can meditate.

Receive the gift each instinct gives you and use it in meditation. Be at home with gathering. Draw nourishment from your hunter. Take strength from your nurturer. Make friends with each of these as they show up to assist you. Do not turn them away as scoundrels; they hold the keys you will need to make your way on the quest. In the myths, when an animal comes and rubs against you in a friendly way, it is at your peril if you chase it away.

Meditation helps you get into the sense of wholeness, where all your instincts are free to play in you. But to stay there in daily life takes some skill. You need to learn to sense your boundaries, get the feeling of your individuality in motion, and move with your rhythms. At first this may seem like pride, arrogance, smugness, uppityness. If so, good. Give it a couple of years to mellow out on its own. Don't rush to be humble; life is humbling enough. See how much arrogance you can get away with. This is how you take care of yourself. You want meditation to be natural, in the service of life. This is what life will do anyway, and if you don't go with nature, then you can make meditation work against nature, a state of inner war rather than healing.

Notice especially what instincts make you say, *Oh yeah!* Finding what we can say yes to without reservation is an important clue in learning to embrace life fully. The instincts you enjoy can teach you how to release yourself into the ones you are less familiar with.

When I was in my teacher training, my whole desire was to stay there in my room, meditating all day every day. I felt that I could be enlightened if I could stay there for just 2 more years. I said *Oh Yeah!* to everything involved in staying in the room. My teacher told me to go home and teach, there are people waiting there for you to bring this knowledge to. Don't stay in your room resting, grooming yourself, thinking you are serving God by hiding out. Go forth.

Later my path led me into doing awareness practices all day, on the job as it were. One of these was listening to the name of God resonating in my heart every waking moment: *Elohim . . . Elohim . . .* This was the elixir I needed that year, and it created in me the sense that I was in an inner sanctuary even while I was out in the world teaching.

With each instinct you may find a different elixir or a different way to reach for the elixir: the best healing touch, the quality of light or music that touches you and restores you like nothing else. Use any and all of your sensory pathways. The key is to allow yourself to enjoy and *do* nothing. That is what allows the rest deeper than sleep, the feeling of safety, and the easy sense that you can handle whatever comes up.

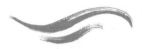

What's Missing?

What instincts don't flow naturally through you? At some point it will be critical for you to identify them and do whatever it is you don't do, refuse to do, or are afraid of doing. It could be anything—you don't play enough, or rest, or explore, or wonder, or nurture yourself.

You have all the instincts, all these abilities, although you will have developed some and neglected others. The people around you often know what you don't do, just as

DON'T DENY

The instinctive tones you deny—either by not giving them time and attention, or because you are afraid of what you feel when you do—follow you around like invisible dogs, barking to get your attention. They can never stop hounding, because they are your life force from which you have cut yourself off.

---

you can see what other people are refusing to do. If you are curious, casually ask around: "What is it I don't do?"

Anytime you have a sense of needing *something*, you might explore that need within yourself. Desires and cravings should be investigated and unfolded, because they often present themselves in disguise. The desire for intimacy may show up as a hankering for ice cream. The desire to take a walk may show up as an interest in a new car. The need to step outside and take a breather may show up as the desire for a cigarette.

When you sense that something is missing, feel where the need is in your body—in your belly, your throat, your heart. Scan your instincts. *Do I need to rest, feed, play, socialize, go shopping?* Test the need by moving with it in some small way, such as taking a short break, stepping out for a breath of fresh air, or scheduling a lunch date.

Whatever is missing or denied will feel taboo when you let it in or start exercising that ability. It may be aggression, acting fierce, protecting yourself, saying no. Or it may be eating with gusto. If you have been dieting for a long time, feeding freely may feel like new territory fraught with horrors.

But, when you do feel more than a few of your instincts alive and vibrating inside you, a quality I want to call the rage for life emerges. I don't know how else to refer to this

LORIN'S NOTEBOOK

TONY AND LUCINDA: OVERCOMING OBSTACLES

Any of the instincts can seem like an obstacle. Take the case of Tony, 28, who works in design. He told me that when he meditates he becomes aware of all the things he wants to change in his apartment. His impulse is to get up and rearrange the room. "I feel restless," he said.

"That's not a problem," I said. "Cherish the impulse to move. If you want to get up, then go with that and get up."

On further inquiry, it turned out that Tony wasn't really at home in his apartment. He would watch TV, but he couldn't shake the feeling that he didn't really like the way things were arranged. When he meditated, his nesting instinct came to the fore. When he indulged it by remodeling the room, which took weeks, he had a new-feeling apartment without having to pack up and move. Then, finally, when he sat still, he felt like the place was his. This was a ritual—his own act of feng shui.

When you dissociate from your instincts or don't honor them when they come up, you impoverish yourself. Eventually the impulses will give up and stop coming to mind. Then it will be that much harder to access them. (At that point you may become attracted to someone who channels these same instincts naturally.)

profound sense of zeal for life. When you come across this in yourself, cherish it and learn from it. I say rage for life in a positive sense, the feeling that *I am a part of nature and I am here to give and receive from the world.* This is a healthy sense of aliveness that leads a meditator out into the world to accomplish her or his goals in harmony with others.

If you are in search of healing, note that usually it is not meditation alone that heals. It is the rhythm of working, eating, meditating, playing, socializing, sleeping, working, eating, and meditating that brings about the higher state of health. Only you can find this rhythm and the clues, hunches, and navigational tips that come to you from all sides and from within.

Lucinda, a mother of three girls ranging from 11 to 17, knew all about nesting. Her whole life was given over to making other people feel at home. When she sat to meditate, she immediately went deep and found rest within her being. But within seconds, she had flurries of thoughts about all the things she had to do. To just sit there, relaxed, felt utterly taboo to her. She nurtured others, not herself. It was very challenging for her to face this, even though in her life she was feeling extremely depleted, chronically tired, and unsatisfied. The reality was that she did have time to take care of herself. Her family did want her to relax, be happy, and thrive. But Lucinda had pushed aside her own needs for so long that she was a stranger to them. Her solution was to take long walks in the hills behind her house, and make meditation part of her outdoorsy wild woman nature. Even after several years of meditation practice, she always prefers to go for a walk or stand in the garden, and then find a place to meditate. Walking is her transition from the life of duties to taking care of herself.

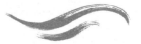

The Instincts in the Sacred Traditions

If you are a Jew, a Christian, or a Moslem, you may have read the Psalms in the Bible. In the Psalms, David goes through a whole series of predicaments—beset by enemies, alone, afraid—but he's also victorious, dreaming, celebrating. If you read them through, you find that all kinds of human emotions and instincts are honored in the Psalms and given their place in relating to God. For example, David sings about his relationship to God in terms of protection—"He is my refuge and my fortress" (Ps. 91:2)—and rest: "He maketh me to lie down in green pastures. . . . He restoreth my soul" (Ps. 23:2–3).

In the Alcoholics Anonymous (AA) 12-step program, step 11 is prayer and meditation. AA is based on spiritual traditions of past centuries, so although it is not overt, its lineage is close to the heart of the Christian meditation tradition. Step 11 describes meditation as a "step out into the sun," a kind of food, light, and fresh air for the soul, as basic a need as having fresh water. Step 11 is a fine piece of writing, full of healthy, instinctive metaphors, and I recommend it to anyone. It suggests that you read a brief prayer very slowly, savoring every word: "As though lying on a sunlit beach, let us relax and breathe deeply of the spiritual atmosphere with which the grace of this prayer surrounds us." The AA approach also recommends self-examination and the self-correcting of errors that takes place during meditation. This review of one's flaws is a classic Christian meditation practice.

If you have ever been around AA people who have meditated for a long time, you may have seen that many of them have a lively, graceful Zenlike quality, completely unaffected and unpretentious and joyful at their own foibles. This is one of the gifts of meditation and of letting the painful self-examination process flow through you: You see your mistakes each day, you see how to correct them, and then you forget about them and live.

The Christian approach, as inherited by AA, sees meditation and self-examination as being directly linked, and in this is more elegant and effective than the generic Eastern approach, which substitutes a guru for your conscience and teaches you that you have a "monkey mind" that jumps around and is a distraction and an obstacle to meditation. This is a self-perpetuation system: The more you block your instinctual

THERE IF YOU NEED IT

You may need to find a sacred context to associate with so you don't feel lonely on your path. Or you may choose to avoid such contact. I know many people of both persuasions.

inner guidance, the more dependent you become on external authorities to tell you what to do.

Another source of extraordinary grace is Thich Nhat Hanh, a Vietnamese Buddhist monk who among other things walked with Martin Luther King Jr. in some of his famous marches. Hanh's teachings are full of instinctive appreciation. In his little book *The Long Road Turns to Joy* he recommends that you meditate on healthy, instinctive qualities as you stroll along in walking meditation:

- **Pay attention with gratitude. Smile inside as you go.**
- **Be aimless.**
- **Have sovereignty over yourself. Walk like an emperor.**
- **With every step you take, a breeze will blow away your sorrow.**
- **Kiss the Earth with your feet.**
- **The path welcomes you.**

In another sacred tradition, Hinduism, one invites God to be present at the puja, or act of devotion, which includes offerings of a seat (asana), water to bathe in, water to drink, food, flowers, perfume, and a cloth. The instincts are each honored in some way, and they relate the one who prays with the life of the universe.

So you see that in some sacred contexts the instincts are emphasized, while in others they are in the background. But the instincts are not coarse. They are the song of life singing you into existence, in an earthy and passionate way.

The instincts are the path you walk, the wave you ride into transcendence. And they are the road back from the quest, the means for connecting your inner life with the outer world.

Let each instinct take what it needs from meditation.

Let each instinct give its gift to your meditation.

Drink, eat, breathe with, wear, bathe in, be massaged by, commune with the elixir of the gift, as you like.

3

Meditation as Healing Attention

The words *medicine* and *meditation* both come from the Indo-European root *med*, which means to measure, to take appropriate measures, to look after, to attend to. There is a musical sense of *med* as well—a measure is also a phrase of music, a beat, so the root also has to do with producing harmony. From the vantage point of etymology, meditation means "paying attention in such a way that harmony is restored." Indeed, meditation is prescribed as medicine in many contexts: to help people recover from stress-induced ailments, to prevent relapses, and to stay out of trouble in the first place.

In its simplest form, attention in meditation means you just become available to yourself. You are just there, witnessing what is going on. The brain, nervous system, and body are a vast symphony. You listen and begin to hear many rhythms, and you realize you are the rhythm. If you sense a disharmony, paying gentle attention will tend to bring it into harmony. If you can feel one part of yourself is out of rhythm with the whole, paying attention will tend to bring about a synchronization of the beat. When you sense that something is missing, an element is needed, your awareness of that need invokes the element. This is healing attention—you are paying attention in meditation in such a way that your own balance is restored.

Meditation is often presented as some otherworldly or spiritual practice, but if you look at the basic technique, you find something very different—that it's earthy, primitive, sensual, rhythmic. Meditation is simply about being attentive to the dynamics of life, to the ebb and flow of breathing, night and day, silence and sound. To meditate, just think of any aspect of nature that you love—the sun, the wind, a mountain, a waterfall, a tree—and cherish all the subtle sensory impressions that come with that thought. For healing meditations in particular, rest your attention in an aspect of how life renews itself: feeding, gathering, resting, fighting, lovemaking, exploring, migrating, building, nesting. Placing the attention on these natural instincts is the basis of meditation techniques known the world over.

As we have already learned, when the body is hurting, pain calls our attention to it. Usually we distract ourselves if we can, for as long as we can, before answering the call. When we just sit there and pay attention to the pain, that is meditation.

Almost everyone I have ever met who practices meditation does so out of a search for healing of some emotional, physical, or spiritual wound or discomfort. If and when you are ready to answer some call and embark on your own quest for wholeness, just remember that the magic of meditation is not connected with any specific meditation technique—rather, it's in the quality of attention that we pay to our lives.

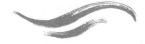

What Happens When You Meditate?

Meditators have been involved in medical and physiology research for many years. Results from these studies have been published in hundreds of scientific journals, including *Behavioral Medicine, Cardiology, Clinical Journal of Pain, Headache, Journal of the American Medical Association* (JAMA), *Lancet, Nature, New England Journal of Medicine, Radiology, Science,* and *Scientific American,* to name just a few. I myself was a subject in a physiological study of meditation at the University of California at Irvine, so some of the blood, breath, and brain waves that have been analyzed are mine. (I still have significant scars on my wrists from catheters that Archie Wilson, one of the meditation researchers, inserted into my veins to measure blood flow during meditation.)

Here now are some of the mind-body findings that support the healing effects of whole body meditation.

THE EMOTIONAL EFFECTS OF MEDITATION

Even if you think you are not an emotional person, you are likely to feel worlds and worlds of emotional nuances during even a 20-minute meditation session. What people report most often are impressionistic images and a sensation of texture that is almost physical, like running your fingers over a woven surface—the emotional texture of your daily life.

You will sometimes find yourself feeling safe and snug during meditation, and at other times you will run through all of the emotions you experienced in the past day or two. Specifically, your body will bring up for your review every emotion that you felt but did not express completely. Whatever your natural responses were during the day that you could not or chose not to express will flow through your body, and you will feel them. If you were shocked during the day on some deep level, then you may cry, shake, shudder, moan, or laugh. Or you may just feel an inward gushing of emotion and show no outward sign.

What happens is often like this: One moment you are focusing on your breath, the next moment you are in the theater of your mind, watching a soap-opera-like scene from your day, and you are noticing feelings you had in your body that you didn't fully appreciate at the time. It could be anything. You might find yourself hearing an undertone of sorrow in your friend's voice, and your heart aches. You could realize that you were jealous of someone but you didn't admit it to yourself at the time. Or, on your mind's screen you might find yourself looking into the eyes of someone you love and realize with a pang that you haven't heard from or reached out to her in a long time—too long.

This catharsis is an inseparable part of meditation. In nature, as in the theater or the opera, all of that drama can intensify the feeling of relief.

THE PHYSICAL EFFECTS OF MEDITATION

Research shows that once you close your eyes to meditate, your body begins to shift into a state of restfulness that is much deeper than deep sleep, and yet you are awake. This level of restfulness brings on a whole set of physical changes: blood pressure decreases, heart rate decreases slightly, breathing rate slows, and muscle tension decreases. The rate of change is startling. Within the first 3 minutes of meditation, oxygen consumption has been shown to drop by as much as 10 to 17 percent; in deep sleep, oxygen consumption drops over the course of hours by only 8 percent or so. Because oxygen consumption is a good indicator of how much work the body is doing, meditation can relax you more than the deepest, most refreshing sleep that you've ever had—and you have access to that feeling in as little as 3 minutes whenever you want.

This and other, similar benefits are side effects of the body just doing its thing. You don't have to tell your heart to beat faster when you are scared, and you don't have to tell yourself to relax and slow down when you meditate. With whole body meditation, you invite the healing instinct to happen, and it happens spontaneously, and a whole world of changes begins to occur within you on all levels. You can usually count on it—within several minutes, the body begins to shift into a state profoundly different from waking, dreaming, or sleeping, but having qualities of each.

In general, you can say that the practice of whole body meditation utilizes Dr. Benson's relaxation response, which is the answer to the body's outmoded stress response. In terms of survival, it gives practitioners an effective way to more quickly recover from fatigue and stress, and training on how to be more efficient at dealing with stressors in the future. For example, if you customize your meditation to address a specific ailment such as asthma, where you'd focus on breathing in the good, soothing air and breathing out the old, bad air, then this may have a more powerful effect.

Of course, meditation isn't as screamingly fast as the stress response; the measurable physiological changes take minutes to show up on a scientist's graphs. Usually it takes a minute or two just to settle in, to get comfortable and get a sense of yourself before beginning. But sometimes meditative relaxation combined with alertness comes to you very fast in daily life, when you need it. The brain is always working very

GET USED TO RAPIDITY

When you meditate, you enter a state in which your body sloughs off stress at a rapid rate. This rapidity is a boon in that we can come home, meditate, have dinner at a reasonable hour, and then get on with the evening. Plus, we need to be able to meditate in the morning before work to prepare for the day.

fast, and when you exercise it with regular meditation, give it a chance to practice its range of motion from utter relaxation to intensity, you'll find you have more—and more surprising—moments of pure zest in life.

Because scientific research has recorded measurable physiological results with meditation as well as with certain yoga techniques and even shamanistic visualizations, these and other healing modalities once considered alternative are now beginning to be worked into mainstream medicine.

THE MENTAL EFFECTS OF MEDITATION

Meditation is a combination of many different states, not one monolithic tone of relaxation. Rather, you'll find you are mentally very quiet at some times and extremely active at other times. The rhythm can be quick—a few seconds of inner silence and then a few seconds or minutes of inner noise. In fact, you can never predict what you will experience from one moment to the next. That's part of what makes meditation interesting and beneficial, but it's also a challenge.

One of the things that throws meditators, beginners and experts, is that meditation only feels like meditation some of the time. The rest of the time it seems like you're just sitting there worrying or making lists. You will find yourself entering states of very deep relaxation, and then suddenly you will recall in detail some time when you were stressed. In your mind's eye you'll see an image, a face, hear a conversation, and in your body you will feel twinges of the stress response. Not the full response, just 1 percent of it, but you will feel your breathing accelerate and your nerves activate. You might find yourself replaying a situation over and over and over in your mind until you can go through it and have no stress response at all, just relaxation.

What is going on here is that your body's survival wisdom has hijacked your meditation time for its own purposes. That's okay. In fact, it's the key to whole body meditation. Your body will use the relaxation and safety of the meditative state to review all the times during the past when you pushed the panic button. Everything that bothered you, all the stressors you encountered—your worries, your undone to-do lists, the promises you have made and haven't fulfilled yet, everything you're scared about— these will come to mind to be dealt with. This gives you the chance to renegotiate your stress response. After all, who says your heart rate has to accelerate and your digestion stop cold because a supervisor walks into the room? Through practice you can convince your body that you are not going to engage in actual physical combat with coworkers at the office or loved ones at home, even if they sometimes set your nerves on edge. This deconditioning will allow you to stay relaxed during your daily life and encourage your natural healing instincts. It's a briefing and debriefing, like soldiers and military pilots go through before and after each mission.

Many forms of psychotherapy are based on this process. Once the patient feels relaxed and safe, then she can talk about her troubles until she feels better—and better able to handle similar problems in the future.

The bottom line with meditation is that you can't rest and relax this deeply without letting go of tension. When you let go of muscular tension, you become aware of what you have been tense about. You are flooded with images, sensations, remembered conversations, and emotions related to what you were afraid, anxious, or worried about.

Stress is a part of life. A lot of it comes from our nerves staying perpetually revved. Even the good things in life have stressful aspects—putting yourself in challenging situations, for instance. Meditation, then, as the opposite of the stress response, is not about eliminating challenge from your life. Rather, it is there to enhance your ability to heal from the wear and tear.

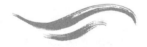

Being with Pain

Pain, we instinctively know, is a signal that something is wrong. Human beings experience not just physical pain, from aching joints or muscles or body systems, but emotional pain and even spiritual pain. Pain calls the attention, and one purpose of meditation is to enable us to answer that call as quickly and as effectively as possible, because we have clearer information about the pain itself, what it means and what it indicates.

Pain narrows the field of focus. Ordinarily when we close our eyes to meditate,

Pay Attention to the Pain

When you meditate, ask the pain what it needs, or ask yourself what you sense it needs. This asking does not have to be in words; simply attend to the pain with a sense of wonder. After all, doctors are called attending physicians because they use their senses to ascertain what the patient needs and then they give it. There is no one "medicine" that everyone needs.

there are thousands of things we could pay attention to. It is like walking into a forest and looking around: Each leaf can be an object of attention, as can each tree or all the trees in the field of view—or the tiniest mote of dust floating in the shafts of sunlight filtering through the branches. When pain calls, however, it exerts a strong pull on our attention, to the extent that it would be an effort to focus on anything else.

There are many nuances to being with your pain, just as there are a million ways to pay attention when you are being with a child, your dog, a horse, a song, or a wide-open landscape. When you engage with yourself in meditation, you continually learn new subtleties of being with yourself. So you are there with your pain, whether it is a heartache, a headache, a pain in the neck, or a pain in the butt. What do you do?

- Be tender.
- Relax into the suffering.
- Give it warmth.

- Give it air, promote circulation.
- If it is too hot, cool it down.
- Give it space.
- Touch, embrace, and contain the pain.
- Inquire: *What are you telling me? What do you want?*
- Be suspicious: *Pain, are you here to distract me from something else, from some greater pain I don't want to face?*

You may need to do all of this and more to deal with your pain. Everyone is different, and each moment of pain we experience may be different in more ways than we have language to describe. The way to start is to simply be with the pain and see what happens. It is similar to being with another person—there is a dance of attention that entails different moves depending on the situation, the mood, how you feel, and how he feels. You can warm your hands by blowing on them, or you can cool them by blowing harder. You can simply listen to someone, or you can laugh with her, challenge her, love her.

One reason that people who are suffering from chronic pain recommend meditation is that the pain that is faced and felt becomes different from the pain you try to block

COMPLEMENTARY MEDICINE

One thing you should never do is avoid medical treatment because you plan on meditating. Meditate in addition to getting regular medical treatment.

(continued on page 122)

LORIN'S NOTEBOOK

ROB: WHAT'S YOUR PAIN LEVEL?

Here is a prescriptive approach to pain relief from longtime meditator Rob Swan. Rob got into meditation to help manage the intense pain he suffers from a debilitating ailment.

"To me, there are three levels of pain. First, there's pain that can be tolerated while one is being completely still. Second, there's pain that one cannot bear for long without moving some other part of the body to distract one from the pain. The third level of pain is so intense that all one can do is put head between legs and try not to pass out.

"Pain in the first level can be lessened with meditation, and meditation can lessen some pain in the second level back into the first. The meditation involves focusing on the pain, wherever it is. If the pain is in the legs, then one would say out loud, 'Pain in legs,' whenever his focus left the pain in the legs. This process of focusing on the pain and bringing the focus back to the pain by saying where the pain is should continue until the pain increases by a substantial amount.

"Then one should say, 'I feel the pain and I let go,' over and over.

"Then one should say, 'I let go of the pain and I get stronger,' over and over. This allows a pressure valve to release, and is done until the pain decreases from its original state.

"The second type of pain can be lessened by moving the part of the body that's in pain very slowly. For instance, if you have a headache, then move the neck very slowly. What you will find very likely is that your body has been attempting to block the pain by tightening muscles. Relaxing the body raises the level of pain in the short run, but in the long run, relaxing the body is the only way to lower pain.

"For most types of pain, if I take 30 minutes to concentrate on it, I can cut the intensity of the pain in half—sometimes I can decrease it much more than that.

"I find it useful sometimes to engage in labeling behavior—to name my thoughts 'thoughts' and feeling 'feelings' (pain is labeled as a feeling). I don't know why this helps—it could be it just gives me something to do. As the meditation progresses, and the mind slows down, and the body begins to relax, I shift to labeling (inwardly) the area where the pain is located. If the pain is systemic, then I just say the various parts of the body as my attention tours through the pain. For example: face, wrist, neck, shoulders, face, elbow, stomach, chest, face, stomach, face, chest, legs, stomach. . . . etc. One should get more and more specific about where the pain is located as the meditation moves on.

"The goal is to have the mind concentrating on two things: identifying thoughts as 'thoughts' and identifying pain by the word that represents where the pain is in the body.

"Doing this provides maximum attention to the pain. During the meditation, the pace at which one labels thoughts and various areas of the body will slow down. As the mind slows, the body relaxes, and the pain increases. With practice, one will learn when enough time has gone by—when enough attention has been given to the pain in order to stop the meditation and observe how the pain has changed."

out or run away from. What usually happens with pain when you meditate is that it gets worse at first, or seems to, because you are focused on it. As your muscles relax, circulation is restored and the pain usually recedes. Here then is the natural instinct to heal in action. Many people discover such processes and never use the word *meditation,* which is fine; you can call the process anything you like, as long as you recognize that it works.

Take the case of Ann, a woman in her early twenties who was getting afternoon headaches at her new job. Finally, she answered the call. "I took a break and went outside and sat under a tree on a bench. When I first just gave myself over to the pain, it felt like it was going to crack my head open. As I sat there and breathed with the painful sensation, it started to throb. It got worse, and I wondered if this was working. Then it got softer. The throbbing turned into a pulse. The sensations shifted into something other than pain. There was a bright light and a high-pitched sound. I opened my eyes after some time, perhaps 15 minutes. There was no more pain, and I had learned something. The pain had taught me about what I was doing to myself, the pressure I was putting myself under. Then each day, when I would first detect the beginning of a headache, I would just pay attention to it a little, and it would go away. After a couple of weeks, the headaches didn't come back anymore. Occasionally, if I am under a lot of pressure, I still get that pre-headache feeling, but I know what to do, and I haven't had a real headache since then."

This example illustrates the basic rhythm of meditation as well as the healing cycle (see "The Healing Cycle" on page 15) at work:

- The call to meditate—there is some need.
- You settle into meditation and encounter obstacles and allies.
- You have a moment of contact with your inner life that changes everything.
- You feel the need to return to everyday life.
- You resume your normal activities slightly transformed.
- This cycle repeats itself again and again, and every half-minute or so there is a mini version that occurs.

Regarding headaches: There is a saying among physicians who specialize in headaches that "Every headache is unique." There are dozens of different reasons people's heads ache, from sinus infections to chocolate allergies to emotional reasons. Always investigate your body and use the best of medical knowledge you have access to when pain lasts or seems to indicate a need for treatment.

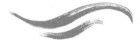

Baptism in the Elemental Elixirs

If you were to go to an alternative healer—a Tibetan doctor, an Ayurvedic physician, or an acupuncturist, for example—he or she might diagnose you by saying you are low on some element or another. The prescription might include herbs, a healthy diet, and a healing meditation to balance your elements. These elements are not the ones mapped out by physics but are rather the phenomenological elements—the ones you encounter directly with your senses as you taste, smell, move through, feel, and look at life. I am talking about luscious, raw experience; no microscopes needed. Each of the elements of air, earth, fire, space, vibration, and water is a different kind of elixir and offers its own gift of healing.

What I suggest you explore in this section are your cravings for each element. Get familiar with the elements, become intimate with them, get used to receiving their gifts. Work your way through the obstacles of awkwardness, fear, and overreliance on

BON VOYAGE

In the past, when sailors would set off on a voyage they would commend their souls to God. The priest may have had a mass for the men and offered them a blessing. Even today, when a ship is launched it is traditional to break a bottle of champagne on the bow—an offering to the gods.

What, for you, is an appropriate way to begin the adventure of meditation? You could go public with your intention—confer with a priest, rabbi, imam, therapist, or guide of some kind and say, "I am going to be starting meditation and would like your blessing." Or, I know people who go to nature for support when they undertake a practice. They spend an afternoon or a day or several days in the desert, mountains, ocean, or forest communing with nature. And there are those whose connection to God is so strong that they need not go anywhere outside themselves or confer with another person— they simply rest in prayer and draw their energy from inside.

The important thing when you begin meditation is to make it a healthy and happy place for yourself right from the start so that you will be motivated to meditate your whole life long, through thick and thin.

one element. You may find that as you feed yourself a more varied diet of elements, your physical health becomes stronger. In essence, in these meditations you are giving your body's self-balancing instincts a chance to play in the fields of gravitation, vibration, air, the fires of life, and water.

Many meditation techniques are combinations of the senses and the elements—pay attention to the sensations of the air as it flows though you. Listen to the sound of a mantra and the feeling of its vibrations in your body as it comes and goes and fades away into silence. Perceive the light that shines on the subtlest level and drink the elixir of it. Visualize yourself sitting with Buddha or Christ and breathe in rhythm with him. Each meditation tradition emphasizes certain combinations of elements, senses, and instincts. In that sense, any particular meditation school is like a restaurant specializing in one style of cooking.

Meditation is sometimes taught as an imaginal journey in which you go to your favorite spot on Earth, or the most beautiful place you can imagine, and be there with all your senses. The key is to give yourself permission to enter that vision with all your senses and let it be utterly alluring, so you'll want to go there. The elixir is the particular combination of senses and elements that makes you feel restored. Right now, can you feel in yourself a craving to be somewhere else? What would that place be like?

Take a breath and let your mind wander and conjure a location so perfect that you would hardly want to ever close your eyes. It could be along a riverbank, in the middle of a desert, on the top of a mountain, standing in the ocean surf, or secluded on a tropical island. You could be by yourself or with others.

If you are at the shore, for example, you could look out over the aquamarine water to the horizon, enjoying the rhythm of the waves and feeling the gentle ocean breezes touching your body as you inhale the vitality-giving air. Feel the warmth of the sun on your skin as you listen to the *shhhhhhhhh* sound of the foam gushing and ebbing on the sand. Turn around and you will find a brook flowing from the mountain, and the water of this stream has magical healing properties. You dip your hands into the water and drink, and it fills you with a wonderful electric feeling, like the best champagne.

GOING SOLO

One advantage of not studying with a teacher is that no one owns you, no one has dibs on your soul, you are not bowing down to someone or some predetermined scheme of things. When meditation is associated with one Indian guru, one Tibetan tulku, and you find out that he has been sleeping with his students' wives, your whole belief in the process can be shattered. If you are in one of the many cultlike meditation groups around that are inflated with a sense of their own specialness and you utter the wrong thought, you may be rejected.

The world is full of people wanting to steal your inner authority. But meditating on your own, in the context of your daily life, and using your senses and your life as your feedback mechanism is a great way to go. It will take you longer in some ways, because person-to-person contact is so useful, but in the long run you are always better off developing your internal guidance first.

Imagery such as this works well, particularly on tape and when you like the speaker's voice, because meditation is so much about the subtle, interior use of the senses. What happens when you do such guided imagery over and over is that you build a pathway to that place, and eventually you won't need the whole intricate process of visualization any more. You close your eyes, take a few breaths in the same appreciative manner you would on that beach, and you are there.

You can see from the way that you relate to the imaginal world that it involves your senses—seeing and hearing and smelling and tasting and feeling—as well as the elements of air (wind, and the breath as it enters your body), earth (sand or mountains or soil), fire (the sun or stars), space (the sense of being uncrowded, of openness stretching out to the far horizon), and water (river or ocean or lake), as well as vibration (an energy that encourages communication and the organization of thoughts). Your particular healing elixir is a unique combination of these elements, designed by your deep spirit to renew you, restore you, and give you the strength to continue on your way.

The elements are intimately related to the instincts (see "Instincts Lead the Way" on page 66). Notice what you have an instinctive craving for, take joy in, feel at home with, and can rest in. In meditation you want to be able to feed, play, hunt, explore, mate, and more to your heart's content. When you find an element you love, revel in it, be massaged by it. Bring all the instincts you know to bear with each element. You will have a tropism for each one—a moving toward it for energy or nourishment.

Get to know each element over time, but to start with, select three of the elements to explore now by doing the explorations suggested at the end of each elemental description. Just 3 minutes of being in the vibration of an element is enough. You want to let your body get comfortable, settle in. Later, come back and explore all of the elements at your own pace.

AIR

Just because something is invisible and apparently weightless does not mean it is insubstantial. Air is matter, and it is attracted by gravity to surround the Earth. That's why it does not flow away into space. It is the nature of air to expand and permeate everything so that the pressure is equal everywhere. Air always does its best to make sure you can breathe; it even permeates the ocean so that fish can breathe through their gills.

The transparency of air teaches us about the transparency of matter. Air does not resist being penetrated by light—that's what *clear* means. When it's clear, you can see light on a distant mountain. When you are meditating on the air element, you may feel simultaneously that you are matter and yet that the light of being can easily pass through you. You can see the light of your soul, or the light of the chakras, or the flickering, fireflylike light of thousands of thoughts shimmering against a background of space.

Always salute the air when you meditate, for it is the stuff of the breath of life. There is nothing greater than to breathe with conscious gratitude. Air teaches you to

A Cup of Air

I like to drink a cup of air at the beginning of meditation. I move my arms in circular slow motion out to my sides, then curve them around in front gathering air-stuff, the magnetism in air, then I bring it in toward my nose and inhale, as if breathing in or drinking in an elixir. It's a move I adapted from tai chi, a Chinese form of movement meditation.

be lighthearted and breezy and to realize the insubstantiality of things. Air refuses to get bogged down with anything that pretends to be too heavy—this it dismisses with an airy wave. When we engage with air, either unconsciously or consciously, it has something to do with circulation.

All your senses inform you about the air flowing in and out of your body 16 times or so a minute. You can smell the air, taste it, sense its motion, and when you breathe out you can feel how the temperature has risen by 10 degrees and is moistened by its passage. The action of breathing, the rhythmic pumping of the lungs, can be felt throughout the body. All this infinitely changing sensory texture is why people can meditate on breath for years and be led ever deeper into appreciating life's mysteries.

Explorations: Go sit on a mountain or at the shore or wherever you can easily find the wind. Or just imagine you are in such a place. Bathe in the wind and let it caress you (Benjamin Franklin was famous for taking air baths). Let the wind blow away your cares. Be groomed by the wind, loved by the wind. Listen to what the wind has to say.

If you find a place of heaviness in your body during meditation, just be with it for a while as it is. Then begin to be aware also of the lightness of air, the exquisite touch of air, the way air gently penetrates everything. These ethereal yet fleshly qualities may be a soothing balm for that heavy place. Let these qualities "be present" in the vicinity of the heaviness, so that at last when that part of you sighs, on its next breath it can breathe in this balm.

Lie on your back and gaze upward into the immense circle of the sky. If it is daytime, accept that you are living in an ocean of air that goes up for miles. If it is night and you can see the stars, appreciate them for generating oxygen and breathing it out into space.

During meditation or anytime when you are breathing, recognize that you are feeding on air. One way of exploring air during meditation is to have a very faint pleasant smell, so faint you can hardly tell it is there, in the room with you when you are meditating. From time to time during your meditation, come to your sense of smell and inhale. Can you detect the smell? I like to meditate in the early morning hours before dawn. Outside the house are various kinds of flowering plants that open and close at different times. As I am meditating, the night-blooming jasmine fades into other scents.

EARTH

The earth is the ground we are standing or sitting on. Being aware of our relationship with the earth is the foundation for spiritual practice.

Earthiness is the quality of embracing all life's functions and being uninhibited and natural ourselves. In whole body meditation you are seeking to bring an earthy enjoyment of life into your meditative experience. When you walk, feel your feet touching, kissing, caressing the earth as a lover. Pay attention to your legs and notice the way your bones are designed to hold you up by resting in their own structure. The bones are made strong by gravity, by moving appropriately in the earth's gravitational field. With each step, the small stresses of walking tell the bones to make themselves stronger. Astronauts lose 1 percent of their bone for every month in zero gravity.

The earth calls us through gravity. When you sit in meditation, let gravity pull you down deep into the chair. Gravity is a massage, pulling some parts of you down while aligning you. You have a gravitational sense, the vestibular sense or inner ear, that continually tells you your relationship with gravity and coordinates in the brain information from the eyes and joints.

Be aware of sitting on the earth. Find out where the different directions are—north,

THE GIFT OF GRAVITY

Gravity is a total paradox. When you let yourself sink into the earth, after a while you will feel yourself flying, levitating. Surrendering to gravity teaches relaxation and levity. You can breathe with gravity, rest in it, play with it, be massaged by it, and excrete into it. When you are utterly relaxed and in meditation, it is as if the unwanted old stuff, old woes, sinks into the earth.

south, east, west—from where you are sitting. Look at a photograph from space of where you are. Be aware of the world beneath you. Put your attention in your tailbone and notice what you can sense there. Be aware of the horizon, the earth curving away.

Explorations: Sit perfectly still while tipping your head about a half-inch to the left, then to the right, then forward, then back. By noticing the interaction of your body and gravity in this way, you learn what's up with your posture. Gravity will teach you how to sit upright, because you can tell by the weight whenever your body is out of alignment. Move your head in a tiny orbit—no more than an inch, and slowly. You will find a speed that is delicious. Get a circle going so it continues of itself. Allow the speed to slow, so that you can't tell whether you are moving or not. This exercises the vestibular sense in combination with the motion sense.

Now stand up. Close your eyes, lean forward from the hips, and oscillate from side to side, exploring slow motion. Movements such as these can be a bridge into and out of meditation. The sensations are usually fleeting and subtle, but over time you will learn to track them, learn from them, be entertained by them. Move about very slowly in any manner that pleases you and notice where your center of gravity is. Keep coming back to this simple exploration again and again for a few minutes each day. Then sit, or rather let gravity pull you toward the earth and enjoy the feeling.

FIRE

Fire is an interaction of elements such that they give off energy and produce heat, light, or both. In your body, each cell is a little furnace, burning oxygen and sugar to

DRINK THE SUN

Light can be nourishing. We can drink in colors with our eyes and our skin; the sunlight we absorb brings in vitamin D. Children who are always covered up outside can suffer from vitamin D deficiencies. The light from the sun stokes the green plants, which convert sunlight and earth substance into food. When you eat the food, any food, the energy you get is really reclaimed sunlight.

In 1969 I had a garden and grew carrots for juice. One day I found myself walking outside and offering up a glass of the juice to the sun, then drinking it. This is the primordial movement of drinking the elixir, and I think it has a real, physical effect. Food offered in this way can taste significantly better.

stay alive. The body maintains a temperature of almost 100 degrees. That's hot. With each inhalation, you stoke the fire. The smoke, the excess carbon dioxide, is carried away with every outbreath.

In the outer world, fire includes light in all its permutations—color, the textures you see, and the source of light, which is usually some kind of fire. If you are reading by electric light, that is a kind of fire, and somewhere there is a fire burning in a power plant to provide the electricity.

Light is there, seen or unseen. Fire is always there as long as the flame of life is burning. Be warmed by the fire of life, feel it pulsating, and delight in the steadiness of its flow. You can hear the steady hiss of the flame; indeed, some mantras are effective reminders of what the flame of life sounds like.

The fire element is quick, radiant, impulsive. Fiery people are said to be intense, lively, vivid in their imaginations, and brilliant.

Explorations: Sit in a comfortable place, inside or outside, and rest your eyes somewhere. Usually when we are looking, we actively look out. It is as if we reach out into space with our awareness. This time, be aware of the light coming to you. Let the back of your eyes be open and feel yourself receiving light. Let your whole body be open to and appreciative of light. Then close your eyes and enjoy the memory of light.

Go outside and appreciate the sun for 10 minutes. Take a brief sunbath, as naked as you can be given the circumstances. Feed on the light, let it soothe you, massage you, energize you, calm you. (Do not look directly at the sun; it is too powerful.) Then go inside and sit somewhere or lie down. Savor the aftereffects, the afterglow of the sun.

Another time, light a candle and place it before you and watch it for a while, then close your eyes and meditate. Simply be aware of the candle from time to time and realize that each of your billions of cells is a tiny flame, like a candle or a miniature sun. Candles are great teachers in that they tend to pulsate—that is part of their charm. The pulsating light is a great treat when you sense it in meditation.

As part of your meditation warmup, reach upward with your hands into the space above your head. Pause there for half a minute. Then bring your hands down and rest them, but leave your attention in that space, which is maybe 18 inches above the head. Up here is what is called the soul star, an energy center like the heart is an energy center, only this one is above the body. It has a radiant, starlike quality; it is cool fire, which you may perceive as blue-white light. When you attune to it someday, you may feel as if the sun is shining on you even as you are sitting in the dark. Until then, why not make the soul star reach part of your opening meditation ritual?

SPACE

Space is the element in which all the other elements play. It may seem empty, but it is not; there is always a subtle texture to space somehow. Space is full of something, and fertile. Besides just providing room for things to happen in, space is friendly.

Become aware of the space around you. Appreciate how good it is to have all that space between you and the walls, the roof, other objects, and between your abode and the next. Notice that you have preferences for space. You might like your home to be farther away from your immediate neighbor's, but would you want it to be 1,000 miles away? The Earth has a tremendous amount of space around it, and it re-

OPEN HEART

Arriving at a spacious area can be a huge relief, but some people are scared of it at first because they can sense their boundaries changing. When you walk up a hill or mountain and come to a vista, there is a palpable expansion of the heart. You can actually hear this feeling being vocalized again and again if you stand at a tourist's scenic overlook, where you will hear people say *"Ahhhh"* all day long.

quires that much—that's the appropriate distance from the sun and the other planets.

Become aware of the space inside your body. As you breathe, feel how it is the space in your nose that allows the air to flow. Open your mouth and feel around with your tongue. The space in your mouth, down your throat, and into your belly is what allows you to take in nourishment. Your upper torso has a large amount of space, called your lungs, that allows for air to flow in and out.

When you are meditating, you may feel that certain areas of your body are calling out to have more space. If there is congestion, if your breathing is restricted in any way, that part of the body will be asking for more space so that the compression can release into expansiveness and flow. There are millions of little signals like this that you will get from your body during meditation. People who live alone in the mountains or forest often experience "livin' large" and do not feel overly condensed. But if you live in a city, you may come to realize that you are holding yourself too small and need to live larger and let yourself inhabit more space. At the same time, in each moment of meditation let it be a possibility that you can melt into space, that any part of your body can melt, dissolve, and become infinite.

Explorations: Be aware of your whole body and how much space it inhabits, how much space there is around it, and then with a sense of that spaciousness, visit with an area of your body that feels restricted, whether it be your chest, your face, your head, your throat. If your head feels congested with too many thoughts or restricted, for instance, meditate on space—the space between things, the space between thoughts, atoms, or leaves on a tree.

Vibration

There is a delightful phenomenon that propagates itself through earth, air, and space. It has the quality of waves, and takes the form of sound, vibration, resonance, pulsation, and harmony. I feel that this phenomenon deserves its own status as an element for meditation.

When we hear speech in the outer world, we usually do not process it as vibration; instead, we interpret the words to get their literal meaning. During meditation, however, we free up attention to simply enjoy thoughts and emotions as waves of vibrations moving through the body, like music. Some people are just naturally more in tune with this element and drink deeply of it. They move in it, breathe with it—we call them vibrant personalities.

The Spice of Life

If meditation were purely mechanical, then the instructions for incorporating vibration into your meditation would be so simple. However, I have found through in-depth interviews with mantra meditators that when you begin being with sound by rote, you sometimes stay in that mode, year after year after year, like a hypnotic drone. I was astounded when I started interviewing transcendental meditation teachers, yogis, and other meditators who just dutifully repeated their mantras over and over without letting them change, become jazz, or disappear into the sacred silence.

TONGUE *UN*-TIED

I often suggest to people that they should explore the vowel sounds of their native tongue and of any other language they might know. Just roll the sounds around and develop a taste for them, so to speak. In meditation, when people are exploring their preferences for the tones of vibration, for sound, they tend to choose:

1. *ah*	**3.** *am*
2. *oh*	**4.** *e-e-e*

Once you pick the central sound, you can add a consonant or another vowel at the beginning or end.

If you like *ah*, you could explore also *bah*, *jah*, *dah*, *ma*.

With *oh*, you can add almost anything: *bo*, *ko*, *mo*, *lo*, *so*, and on.

If you like *am*, you could explore *gam*, *lam*, *kam*, *ram*, *sam*, *jam*.

And *e-e-e* can be combined with any of the others.

It usually takes about 5 minutes for a person, just playing around, to begin to develop a taste for this sound or that. You use these sounds all the time if

When you meditate on sound, you can listen to the waves within the sound, the up and down of it; you can feel the rhythm of a sound; you can focus on the resonance as it touches your internal organs; or you can listen to the way the sound comes on and then fades into the silence between thoughts. All of these nuances are there to be observed and enjoyed when you listen to even the simplest sound inside yourself during meditation.

you speak, or think, in just about any human language. But unless you are a doo-wop singer (singing backup: *"O-oh, yeah . . . "*) or a yogi, you may not have ever awakened your sense of preference for sound, as you have for foods, music, and movies.

It is well worth your while to explore sound and then go to the classical mantras. You will appreciate how utterly rich they are. The names of God in any religion are so incredible if you are really listening to resonance, that you could happily sit in a room for years just listening:

"Allah . . ."	*"Jahveh . . ."*
"Ram . . ."	*"Ishvara . . ."*
"Elohim . . ."	*"Emmanuel . . ."*

Play with, rest in, explore, feed on these sounds. Your sensibility will evolve. As you get used to the resonance, the sound will at times come from everywhere in your body. As you sit there, it is as if you are within Allah, within God, and He is vibrating within you.

The spoken voice is a breath that is shaped by vibration. Sound that is heard internally, as when you are listening to the thought of the sound *ah*, are a subtle vibration also. There are infinite nuances of these sound-thoughts. The main thing is to enjoy yourself and develop your taste for sound. Play with sound, bathe in it, be massaged by it, purified by it, groomed by the sound. Eat or drink of sound. Let sound be nourishing to your soul.

Explorations: Explore the sounds of language. Which ones are nourishing, soothing, stimulating, restful, or sensual? Be with the vowels *a-e-i-o-u* and sometimes *y*, and also *mmmm, nnnn, shhh, ttttt,* and every other consonant.

Make a gentle sound of *ahhhhhhh* out loud. Do that for a minute, right now if you want. Then whisper it. Then close your mouth and make the sound so that it vibrates your mouth, tongue, and lips. Explore the vibration and resonance. Now think the sound *ahhhh* in your mind without feeling it in your vocal chords. Let it be a thought.

You also might want to listen to any of the world's great chanting or choral music. It is hard to think of a culture that does not have beautiful chanting. Put a chair between the speakers of your stereo and listen. Breathe with the chanting. Lie down on a sofa. Go to concerts, churches. Ask a friend who knows chanting to chant for you. Bathe in the sound and then let there be silence and savor what happens. There are also CDs filled with natural sounds that you can bathe in, drink in, be massaged by: the sounds of oceans, rivers, waves, and the wind through the trees.

WATER

Water is the most plentiful element in our bodies, accounting for most of our weight. Our bodies are about 70 percent water, and water is amazingly heavy for something that is only two hydrogen atoms and an oxygen atom. Carry a gallon of something and feel how heavy it is.

In the outer world, water circulates continuously in rivers, pipes, showers, faucets. The oceans are water, and the fire of the sun heats them, evaporating huge quantities that fall back to the ocean and onto the continents as rain. We live our entire lives within this cycle of water eternally flowing.

In metaphor, something that is watery has the connotation of being watered down, weak, or bland. But the Taoist meditators point out that water is strong; it can wear away the hardest rocks. It is good to be like water—ever flowing.

The blood in your body is mostly water, and it circulates in arteries that branch into ever smaller vessels until every cell is bathed in blood. Honor the blood flowing in your body. It carries the air and the fuel that your cells burn. Meditation can feel like the free circulation of liquid, like a shower or bath, or like drinking water when you are thirsty.

Explorations: As a preparation for meditation, take a shower and let the water drum on your head and massage your skin. Or go to the ocean and mingle with the waves. There are many people who just are not comfortable meditating inside at home. They only really enjoy meditation when they are outdoors in nature, preferably by water in some form—a lake, waterfall, ocean, river, stream, or spring. Interestingly, the image of still water is not appealing for some people; they want to feel like a waterfall, streaming and gushing. This makes sense because the circulation system of the body is not lakelike but moving, gushing.

You might explore having a bowl of water nearby when you meditate, or a glass of drinking water. Either before or after meditating, raise a cup of water and drink of it as if it were the elixir of life.

As you can see, the elements are entertaining. Exploring them is about enriching your experience, so that even when you are sitting still, apparently doing nothing, you are exploring subtle aspects of what it is to be alive.

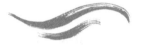

Essential Meditation Instructions

Because the ability to meditate is built in, it can happen spontaneously, as when you sit on a beach listening to the ocean or on the side of a mountain gazing at the horizon. To consciously invoke a state of meditation, the basic procedure is not complicated: Essentially, you just pick something beautiful to focus on gently, and when your mind wanders, return to that focus; continue this for 20 minutes or so.

The idea that meditation could be this simple has been discovered, lost, and rediscovered for millennia. Meditation is somewhat like food preparation: you can just pluck a piece of fruit or a vegetable from the tree or vine and eat it; you can slice it, or you can cook elaborate meals. It can be as straightforward or complicated as you desire. Many people love to make up rules that make meditation difficult—sit cross-legged so that your knees hurt and your feet go numb, and try to not think. Go to any bookstore and glance through the meditation texts and you will find rules about cultivating the proper attitude of submission to the guru, being celibate, eating vegetarian, and doing elaborate visualizations and concentrating really hard. Each rule probably worked somewhere, for somebody, at some stage of his or her development.

The rules I am presenting here are designed to support you in being elegant in your approach to meditation. Elegance means "grace in movement and style." In science, elegance means "the simplest description or set of steps that solves a problem."

In meditation, grace comes from letting your instincts guide you, and using something you love as a focus, so that you want to pay attention to it and rest with it.

To develop a focus for meditation, you combine an element, a sense, and an instinctive tone.

Choose a soothing and beautiful image or sound from nature or your religious tradition; or a sensuous quality of your breath (see page 56). Selecting the focus is very individual because you want it to be something you enjoy being with. There are an infinite variety of choices. You might want to take a breath right here and read the next couple of paragraphs slowly.

Select an **element** to focus on: water, light, earth, air, space, vibration. With water, you could be thinking of a river or feeling the flow of blood through your body. With air, you could be enjoying your breathing. With vibration, you could be listening inwardly to a sound, such as the remembered sound of a waterfall, or one of the names of God.

You select a **sense** to focus with: hearing, touch, smell, vision, motion, balance. Usually one sense will be primary and then, with experience, all the other senses come into play. For example, you might be feeling the motion of your muscles as you breathe as well as smelling the air and sensing its temperature.

Then select an **instinctive tone** to favor as you are meditating. You may prefer meditation to feel like a bath, or hunting, or exploring, or wondering, or communing. Or you may prefer it to have the quality of grooming, like a massage or sex. You may like meditation to feel playful, or like a big adventure, or like a journey to your inner spiritual home. These are all instinctive tones.

As you explore and play with meditation, your experience will get richer and more interesting as you find the elements, senses, and instinctive tones that engage you the most. You will discover that they will combine and recombine endlessly. You are in essence giving the body permission to meditate while providing a good atmosphere for the process to happen in.

To the extent that you need emotional or physical healing, you will discover specific cravings for what to focus on and how to focus. As you relax you will find that your body actively calls out for this or that kind of attention. Let these cravings be your guide.

Because you will tend to resist cravings that are out of the ordinary for you, over time you need to learn to love a little something in each of the elements, senses, and instincts. You probably already do love something in each; to find out what that is, you simply need to explore.

Begin with something simple, and as you meditate with that focus, your body will give you information about how to modify the focus to make it more interesting. In this way you will learn what you need to as you go along, and your body will modify the flow of meditation to suit your needs. Remember: Meditation is a whole body process that is coordinated by your instinctive self.

LORIN'S NOTEBOOK

SHERRY: THE MANY FACES OF MEDITATION

A couple of years ago I was standing in the self-help section of a bookstore. A woman walked in and asked at the information desk, "Where can I find a book on meditation?" The staff person, Sherry, said, "That is really complicated. There are books on meditation all over the store. There are some in Eastern Religion, of course, but they are also in the Western Religion and Christianity sections. Over here in Alternative Health, and also in Women's Health, are dozens of books that have instructions on how to meditate. In Self-Help there are many more with approaches to meditation that different psychologists have worked out. In the Sports section there are books on yoga that have chapters on meditation. Over there in Addiction and Recovery, quite a few of the books are about meditation. What approach to meditation are you looking for?"

Sherry's exposition wasn't complete, actually. She didn't mention, or did not know, that in the Sexuality section there are books on how to meditate as part of lovemaking; in the Biography section there are books detailing the writers' experiences in meditation; in the New Age section there are many approaches to meditation; and in the Outdoors section there are books on developing tracking, hunting, and other meditation-related instincts.

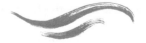

Keep Returning to Simplicity

Meditation is simple; it's your experience that is complicated. That's why you need these essential meditation instructions—to make you fully aware of how meditation works in you and, more important, how it *feels*. The skills of meditation are very much like learning to listen to music, enjoying the relationship between the beat and the melody—only you are the music. The life flowing through you is the melody, and your physical structure—your heart, your lungs, your muscles and bones—is the instrument it plays. You learn to meditate by exploring the body, and the rhythms you discover teach you about yourself.

What happens when you are hungry or sexually aroused, for example, is very complicated if you look at all the bodily systems involved. You can have an infinite variety of experience with eating and with lovemaking. With meditation, you can add layers of complexity, and sometimes that's useful and necessary. Aristotle said, "Nature operates in the shortest way possible." Kepler said, "Nature loves simplicity, it loves the unification." And Einstein said, "Everything should be made as simple as possible, but not simpler."

The reason you will need to add some layers of complexity is to match your individuality—your unique life experience and your particular healing needs. Part of the quest for wholeness is to find what works for you and then bring it back for use

LORIN'S STANDARD MEDITATION FORMAT

1. Sit comfortably in an upright posture. Reach your arms up over your head; then bring them down and out in front of your chest; then slowly bring your hands in until they touch your chest. Then rest your hands in your lap.

2. Wait until you feel like closing your eyes. Until then, simply enjoy your breathing.

3. When your eyes close, continue to enjoy your breathing for 2 to 3 minutes. You can notice any combination of the texture, rhythm, temperature, smell, touch, sound, or any other sensory quality of your breathing.

4. Find your own way to be grateful for breath, to express *This breath is the breath of life* or *This breath is a gift from God*. Your way could be a prayer, a thought, or simply the feeling of gratitude. Be with this gratefulness for a short while.

5. Gently cultivate an interest in your focus, which could be any aspect of breath, a mantra, a prayer, a visualization, or a sensation of motion in the body.

6. Take a "Bring it on!" attitude to engaging your sensations, emotions, and thoughts. Even when outer noises attract your attention, don't be concerned. Don't put any pressure on yourself in any way to perform or have a specific experience.

7. When thoughts come, accept each one as a gift from your instinctive inner intelligence and accept the energy, alertness, and insight it brings.

8. Toward the end of the meditation, rest for a minute with some great thought or quality you are seeking to develop in your life, such as harmony, love, inspiration, power, strength, relatedness, or God consciousness.

9. At the end of the meditation, sit still for at least 3 minutes and up to 5 minutes. Then move just a little. Perhaps have a closing ritual in which you sweep your arms very slowly around to your sides, and in toward your heart.

in your everyday life. In the outer world, people travel far and wide to find the right meditation instructions. Since the late 1960s my friends have gone to places like India and Burma and have come back a year or two later, maybe ravaged by hepatitis, amoebic dysentery, and typhus but having met a guru. Many of them finally found their inner pathways while sitting in some ashram. There they connected with the particular context—and maybe stench—that made them feel, *Now I can look inside.* Some people, on the other hand, can find their inner pathways without traveling in the outer world.

NOTES ON "MINDFULNESS"

I don't know of a more boring way to talk about paying attention than to use the term *mindfulness*. I find it hard to believe that if Buddha spoke English he would have selected the term, which is a translation from Sanskrit. (Simple *fullness* is better.)

This is heretical thinking, of course, but I suggest that you approach meditation with an intent to invoke *sensuality*. After all, when you pay attention, you attend with the senses, whether it be through ears, eyes, or some other sensory organ. Maybe it depends on the nature of your need. If you are overly emotional, you might want to shoot for mindfulness—it's the calmer way. But if you are only too good at controlling yourself, then go for sensuality.

The intricacy is in selecting what you want to focus on. Select a word and repeat it easily in your mind. Find an aspect of your breath you enjoy. The texture of the air as it flows in and out. Rest your attention in that sensation. Imagine the most beautiful vacation spot in the world. Go there in your mind and enjoy it through all your senses. Smell the air, see the light, feel the nature of the place, eat something exotic and wonderful, and pay attention to the sensations of your body. You basically create a situation that invites meditation, and then take it as it comes.

As you explore, you will find yourself adding things to your procedure that help. You might find that you enjoy meditation more if you clean up your room first. You might download the top layer of your mind onto a piece of paper—meaning that you go over your to-do list in your mind and then write it all down. Or you may feel better during meditation if you exercise first.

With all these things, there is no substitute for exploring and seeing what works. The world is full of people who will tell you, on great and hoary authority, that this thing or that thing is essential. You have to bow down to this statue of a Buddha first; you have to salute the four geographical directions and utter the proper hymn. A friend of mine, a yoga teacher, called recently and told me that he was reading a book on yoga in which the world-famous author had written, "The best floor for doing yoga is of dried cow dung." So there you have it. That would be the ultimate way of doing yoga, in this particular yogi's scheme.

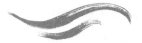

The Need to Accommodate Individuality

From 1970 to 1975 I taught transcendental meditation (TM); after I left the TM organization, through various means it became known that I was a meditation teacher who would just listen. This was because if I wasn't teaching TM, I didn't know what to do.

Los Angeles at that time was a hotbed of meditation experimentation. There were perhaps a thousand TM teachers, plus teachers of every conceivable meditation practice along with all their students. Many people had been meditating intensely for years—sitting for many hours a day, praying without ceasing—and had overloaded themselves. They had the meditator's equivalent of overtraining, what an athlete suffers if she works her body every day with no rest days. If somebody in that situation goes to a teacher in his particular tradition, whatever it is, he will probably be told to meditate more, chant more, eat a stricter diet, be more celibate, and donate more money to the guru. Then the student might look to the alternative health care community. Chiropractors, body therapists, acupuncturists, and homeopathic physicians have many meditators as patients, and as a matter of course ask questions about their meditation techniques.

By a series of coincidences, I became known to these alternative care practitioners as a sort of freelance meditation teacher, so they started referring their clients to me.

The buzz was that you could go to Lorin for a session or two and he wouldn't try to teach you his system or convert you. He would simply help you explore what was happening in your practice.

So I listened. Typically I would pay attention for several hours as these spiritual adventurers would tell me their whole meditation history. At some point, after 45 minutes, an hour, 90 minutes, sometimes 2 hours, they would pause. The room would go silent.

One great thing about working with meditators of any sort is that you can just let a silence hang there. Silence is jazz to meditators. We would just sit there in the silence for a few minutes; then I would ask something like, "What hunches do you have? What feeling do you have about what's next?" They'd always know, and it would almost always be something taboo in the spiritual system they were in.

"Well, to tell you the truth, I really feel I should just stop meditating for a while, or just meditate 5 minutes a day, and start eating meat and maybe have lots of sex."

I'd say, "That sounds like a good idea. Go explore that and see what happens."

Then I would make up a plausible story about how that was a good thing, using New Age terminology. I would say something like, "Your practices have overdeveloped your upper chakras in relationship to your overall system. The craving you have is your inner guidance telling you to strengthen your lower chakras, so that they can support your evolution."

People told me again and again that it was such an incredible relief to talk to

COACHING YOURSELF

When a person is sitting there meditating, she looks just like a person sitting there with her eyes closed. Often, though, there is something extra, a sense of peace about that person.

As a meditation instructor I have learned to use my senses to detect, to some extent, what phase of the meditation cycle someone is in. I can perceive changes in facial muscle tone, breathing rhythm, the pulse at the neck; I can see tiny motions of the body, slight shifts in posture that tell me about how the individual is feeling. More subtly, I can sometimes hear when people are absorbed in silence within, because that gives off a hum, a silent hum such as you can hear in the mountains or in the desert in the wide-open silence.

That being said, meditation is generally invisible behavior. A tennis swing, a sculpture, a chord of music, a note produced by the human voice—all of these are perceptible behaviors that you can get coaching in. Voice coaches and innumerable other teachers can watch you do something and give you correcting instruction. There are thousands of brilliant yoga teachers in the United States—this is something truly great—who over the last 5 to 35 years have been honing their skills and developing Americanized Yoga. They can watch you do a yoga pose and give you good feedback, thus helping you to

someone, because in their entire history of exploration, the teacher would never listen. He would give techniques and then leave them on their own to work out how to do them. Teachers, to many people even today, are mostly inaccessible.

Word-of-mouth referrals were sending me a continuous stream of people who avoid ruining your knees or lower back by doing the poses in the wrong way. Think of a skill, and there are bound to be teachers dedicated to it.

Meditation is a unique and awkward exception in that there is so little to watch that no one can give you really good feedback. There have been the basic methods of biofeedback—such things as the electroencephalogram (EEG), electromyogram (EMG), and galvanic skin response monitoring device (GSR)—but these are not necessarily relevant to meditation. Because of this, good coaching is largely NA (not applicable) to meditation. Being a good coach involves observing someone moment by moment until he gets going, and then being there when he needs you. For the most part in meditation, you're on your own.

An exception to the exception is Transcendental Meditation (TM). In TM training, coaching is given for the first couple of seconds of meditation up to the first few minutes. That is where the main genius of TM is, in my opinion, and how it differs from other meditation traditions. No other technique focuses so intently on what goes on during the first 5 seconds, 15 seconds, 30 seconds, and then 60 seconds of meditation. Because of this, a high percentage of trained TM practitioners get it—perhaps as many as 50 percent of the people who receive TM training will still be meditating every day a year later.

wanted and needed to talk about what was going on with their meditation practice. Even other meditation teachers came, TM teachers, yoga teachers. The one thing I asked when I was finished listening was that they call me in a few months to a year and let me know how they were doing.

Thousands and thousands, even millions of people attempt meditation every year, and most quit in frustration. Some stop altogether, some go on a search from teacher to teacher, trying this system and that. The failure rate of any one meditation system tends to be appalling. No matter how good the teacher, maybe 80 to 95 percent of the

LORIN'S NOTEBOOK

MANNY: TAKING A MEDITATION VACATION

Manny is 37 years old and had given up smoking not long before a recent session, during which I asked him what he experienced when he meditated.

"A flurry of thoughts. Swirling, flickering images of people I saw during the day, scenes. At first, they all have a feeling of static and tension associated with them. Sometimes, one image will come into focus for a while. I see the face of this gal I work with. We were talking and had to stop before we were finished. The phone rang. What did she want to say? An image of my boss's angry face flashes on the screen of my mind. I feel a cold sensation in my stomach. I want to hit him. I feel my body tense up. Every muscle readies itself to plant a good, solid punch to his face. I relish the sensation. After a couple of minutes, I melt, and sigh with relief. It's like I am far away on a mountaintop somewhere. Then, suddenly, I am looking at my desk, what a mess it is. I suddenly remember a piece of paper I didn't deal with. I had told that person I was going to call him back today. Oh no. Now I am aware of tension in my shoulders, a hot feeling. I sigh. My shoulders want to move around, so I let them. The tension turns slowly into fatigue, a sense of great tiredness. I don't want to carry the world on my shoulders anymore. Then I think I dozed for a while. Every-students drop out eventually. To the teachers inside a particular system, these students simply drop off the face of the earth. They are not on the teachers' radar screens at all. They were unworthy, undisciplined.

I was seeing many of these people just as they were about to quit, and it was highly

thing was blank. When I came to, my mind was totally quiet. I didn't move for a couple of minutes, like when you awaken and don't know where you are.

"Around the time I first started meditating, there were a lot of changes at work, and my job was perpetually at risk. I had been living in a state of siege for months. I always had a gnawing, uncomfortable feeling of insecurity. One day I decided to try meditating. On a Saturday morning I sat down and did several short meditations of a minute each, then a 20-minute meditation. I meditated again Sunday morning. I didn't notice much during the meditation—just a lot of thoughts and some physical relaxation. It was nothing spectacular. Then on Sunday afternoon I took a walk. Halfway through the walk it occurred to me that I was feeling better than I had in as long as I could remember. My head was totally clear. I didn't have a worry in the world. All my problems seemed trivial. I had the feeling in the pit of my stomach that I could deal with whatever happened. The world seemed beautiful and fresh. When I went back to work on Monday, the feeling stayed with me. It lasted for weeks, until it became part of me, my normal state. It was as if I had a long vacation and came back with a new perspective. People at work were like, 'Did you fall in love? Are you having an affair?'

"That's what people are looking for in drugs, seems to me. But there's no drug that can do that. Winning the lottery and going on a 6-month vacation might."

informative. Often, it really lifted the top of my head. Just sitting there with a person, for example, it was obvious—it would be obvious to any impartial observer, really—that in almost every case where there was a disagreement between the teacher and the student, the student was in the right.

You would think that teachers in spiritual traditions would know better, but apparently many never learned to say to a student, "You know, you are done here. I have given you all I can. Go forth on your adventure with my blessings, and maybe come visit sometime." I hear of a teacher saying something like this only once every few years.

There is an enormous amount of authoritarian mind-control mentality throughout the spiritual teachings of both East and West. It's "My way or the highway," and about 90 percent of the students take the highway. In the ancient past, when these authoritarian systems evolved, they had a monopoly. If you wanted to learn, you had to submit with unquestioning obedience.

From my perspective, the reason for the high dropout rate is that insufficient instructions are given in how to adapt meditation to your own individual needs.

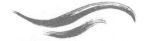

Never Blame Yourself

Since you are reading this book, I have to assume that you are meditating on your own, without a teacher. As we have seen, in the past meditation was almost always part of an organized religious context, practiced by an elite few who had many years of training and supervision before going off to meditate in solitude somewhere. In the modern era, most people who meditate do so on their own. So it is important to know what the obstacles are in advance, so that you don't sabotage your success in meditation.

Most of those I talk to who have given up meditating blame themselves for not being disciplined enough. But that is almost never the case. The people who explore meditation tend to be busier than average, if anything. In talking to people, I find that they are very disciplined in other areas of their lives. No, what gets in the way of meditation is that they lack a bit of knowledge they need to get through the phase they are in. It is as if they came to a door and searched in their pockets and couldn't find the key. No amount of pushing will open the door, either. But some people find that if you just put your hand on the door, touch it, then release the pressure, it opens by itself. This book is about those little findings, what people have figured out that works in applying the ancient wisdom of meditation to modern life.

Meditation techniques are all in the public domain. Thousands of years ago the ancient meditators mapped out tens of thousands of different techniques and formulated them into an oral literature that was chanted and handed down through the meditation traditions. Taken as a whole, the collected wisdom of meditation is a vast ocean of information. The technique you need, the approach or combination of styles you will thrive on, is probably written down somewhere or alluded to. The problem is that 99.99 percent of this information is oriented to the needs of "meditation specialists," virtually all of whom were men who lived celibate lives in temples, monasteries, and other religious contexts. They took other vows besides celibacy—those of poverty and total obedience to their superiors in the order, for instance. Their needs were and are quite different from the needs of people who live in what we call the real world.

The challenge is to find how a modern person, in the midst of her life, can add the blessed sanctuary of meditation to her day and learn to handle all the openings and healings that occur. And even though this common-sense savvy is starting to get around, and there are more and better meditation teachers available, what works for you will still be your unique solution. The tiny adjustments you make here and there while meditating are where you are likely to find the keys.

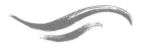

Obstacles

One particular woman comes to mind who encountered an aspect of healing she didn't like, and so she quit. Jane was a single mother of two who worked to support herself and her children. She had a good time meditating and felt very relaxed afterward; the only problem—she usually fell asleep during meditation. The sleep was so deep, "I felt like I was in a coma, I couldn't move," was how Jane described it. This is a typical obstacle that you can encounter: If you are sleep deprived, you will usually fall asleep in meditation. Jane had a big sleep debt, as working mothers often do, and it may have taken 20 hours of extra sleep to get her through it. Then, not only would she be able to meditate, but she would have felt fantastic.

The reality was that Jane had to juggle work and kids and she just couldn't figure out how to get more sleep. I have worked with many people in this situation and often what is going on is that late night, after the kids go to sleep, is the only time they have to be alone and do their own thing. Their entire day, from the time they wake up until then, is go-go-go and completely given over to other people's needs. This is the only time, this hour or two, when they can just enjoy life. The idea of going to bed early, then, seems like too big a sacrifice, too much to give up. (Another woman perhaps could have helped Jane work this through better than I.)

I met Jane at a party years later, and she reminded me about her sleeping during meditation. By then she had developed a perpetual wrinkle in her forehead, the kind you get if you are trying to keep your eyes open.

The stories of Jane and Phyllis (see "Phyllis: Refusing the Call" on page 20) are examples of very common meditation experiences. But please do not think that because I included a success story about a single man (see "Steve: The Journey Fulfilled" on page 54) that women are unlikely candidates for meditation. In fact, the opposite is true. The entire time I have been meditating, from 1968 until now, most of the groups

(continued on page 162)

GOING BEYOND BARE ATTENTION

Some meditation traditions deliberately aim to dissociate attention from instinctive richness. Bare attention, or simply witnessing, is called for sometimes, but meditators who overemphasize this as technique can become overly calm and also devitalized and boring.

I have always been extremely revitalized by meditation, but I fell into the trap of monomania in my own way, and it cost me years of suffering.

Many years ago I received a heart meditation technique from my teacher, who was of the warrior caste in India. It was the classic yoga technique of placing the attention in the anahata chakra, the feeling and energy center located in the area of the physical heart. This was a very powerful experience for me, and initially I was delighted with the feeling of vibration in my chest, and the sense of flow. When I went back a week later for a checkup, I told my teacher my experiences and he looked at me, scowled, and said, "Fine, but when the road gets rough, stay with it," and that was the end of the discussion. He was a tough, no-nonsense guy, and his attitude always was to tough out whatever happened.

For months I enjoyed the nuances that the technique added to my meditation and to my life, but after about a year I began to have an ache in my heart that started as a barely there sensation and grew to be the center of my world. I did not have the language then to say what it was, but it felt just like a heartache. It was as if I was lonely but didn't experience the emotion, I only felt the physical sensation of ache. I attended to the ache for hours every day in meditation, and it rose and fell, shifted and changed in innumerable ways, but it always returned to being an ache like loneliness.

The problem was that my attention was so bare, so totally accepting of sensation on its own level, that I did not learn from the ache. I did not inquire broadly enough, or let attention be called into other tones such as hunting and exploring for what would have helped the ache. I did not communicate and tell anyone, "I am lonely."

I *did* let the ache take me into the God instinct, and I had many long days completely alone, singing love songs to God in English and Sanskrit. I would mark out weeks on my calendar to be in silence, and I would go to a completely isolated beach I knew of and walk there for hours without seeing another person. Then I would sit on the sand and meditate hours more until the sun went down behind the ocean.

It took me years to realize that the ache was calling me out into the world and to connect with people in ways other than just teaching meditation. I was sitting there in meditation, witnessing the ache, giving in to it fully on the level of detached awareness, but I wasn't answering its call. I was not doing anything to soothe the ache, because traditionally meditators learn to just stay with a pain and not try to change it in any way. That was fine as far as it went, but I was overdoing that one tone.

The information I needed was not overtly stated in the teachings of yoga or meditation, although it was there as part of the hidden structure. It was also common sense: Follow your heart and speak from the heart. I know now that I delayed my healing for years by not following this call and letting my skills of attention become more richly nuanced.

and classes I have been in have been 60 to 75 percent women. No matter where I go in the United States or Canada, most of the meditators are women. Until recently, the vast majority of meditation teachers were men, but it seems like that is changing. Fortunately, the more women meditation teachers there are, the easier it will be for women to find their voices and figure out ways through such challenges. It's possible that being the mother in a large family these days (four is considered large now) is more difficult than running four pharmacies. There are many secrets to be unfolded here that women will learn and teach one another.

These secrets, about how to make meditation work in your particular life, are hinted at in meditation teachings, but they do not really belong to meditation. Meditation is, after all, just a condition of being intimate with your deepest self, or more accurately, with all your many selves, while in a state of utter relaxation. It is a bit like lying in bed with your lover after orgasm. If you are really tired, you will sleep; if you are sad, you might cry; if there is an obstacle to intimacy, you will be angry; if you are worried, you will want to talk about it. How to handle all of this is something you can learn while meditating, but you learn it from yourself.

Keep in mind that longtime meditators and meditation teachers are not necessarily very good at these skills of intimacy. Very often, meditation teachers are people who were terrified of intimacy and went into meditation for healing, and now here they are. Everyday people who live rich lives and don't have time to spend years learning to be a teacher are often much more skilled at handling emotions than are their teachers. The essential teachings about accepting what the human heart has to go through to un-burden itself of past hurts and open up to life again are everywhere—in literature, art, music, theater, dance, religion, therapy. I see all the teachings in Judith Krantz novels. It's all there in close friendships. There is nothing in meditation that is not common sense, and the truths meditation has to say are often said better, with more juice, else-where. Meditation is nothing if not being a good friend to yourself.

The difference, what is special and valuable about meditation teachings, is that they tend to be oriented to how to handle this exact experience while you are meditating. Phyllis and Jane got stuck in their meditation because there was something about life they didn't know, or something they did not want to sacrifice in order to meditate. Phyllis didn't want to risk getting into her anger; she had seen women tear up their fam-ilies in their righteous rage, wounding everyone with their claws, themselves most of all. Jane didn't see how she could invent another couple of hours in the day, as if she were a magician who had control over the sun. In each case, the problem was not with meditation—they just didn't like the way that their healing presented itself.

With both Phyllis and Jane, what happened when they meditated was that they got in touch with their needs, and their lives were not about the fulfillment of their needs. These were deep, aching needs because they had been pushed away for years while they put other people's needs first. Phyllis pushed her bad feelings aside and made life work for her family; Jane pushed her need for more rest aside and tended to her job and her family.

Any need that we have that goes unmet for a long period of time tends to become

DON'T SPANK YOUR MONKEY MIND

Much of the literature on meditation amounts to a continual whine about how thoughts come and bother the poor meditator. An immense arsenal of mental weapons is proposed for killing, squashing, inhibiting, blocking, maiming, minimizing, and deleting thoughts. This suggestion comes mainly from monks and yogis sitting cross-legged in their cells, trying to not go crazy thinking about women, wine, and song.

When you accept the opinion that the thoughts that come to you during meditation are just noise, a product of your jumpy "monkey mind," you miss out on valuable inner guidance. Many meditators unfortunately have learned to block out their inner voices. They shout them down with their difficult techniques, rigid belief in the infallibility of their gurus, or obsession with vegetarianism. It is not that difficult, really, to lock your conscience in the closet; people do this all the time in the waking state. When meditators do this, they often get some peace of mind, but there is also a deadened, clueless aspect to them, as if they are heavily medicated. I have often heard this commented on by alternative health practitioners, who see a lot of this type of meditator.

When you reprimand your "monkey mind," you blot out many of the subtle, instinctive clues from your body. The alternative health practitioners have

isolated from the body by a barrier of psychic callus. In order to survive, we often turn against our own needs—for rest, for comfort, for attention—as if they were an enemy. Sometimes a neglected need becomes "infected" by being cut off from circulation. So when at last we let the feelings flow, let circulation be restored, it is like lancing a boil.

mixed feelings about this, because it is good for business. The more meditators block their intuition, the more they will be reliant on acupuncture,
herbs, chiropractic, and other health care systems to keep them tuned.
In other words, you go to someone and you pay them to honor your intuition
for you.

This may sound like an obscure hazard of meditation, but it really is quite
common. Since I began meditating in 1968, I have always known people who
take up meditation, thrive for a while, and then start slowly disintegrating
over time as they gradually cut themselves off from their common sense and
impose more and more externally generated rules on themselves. Without in-
tending to, they find ways to make meditation, yoga, and health food into un-
healthy activities. For many years I accepted the standard, dismissive
explanation for their symptoms so pervasive throughout the meditation and
alternative health communities: "They are just purifying, getting rid of toxins."
After I interviewed quite a few people in this situation in the late 1970s,
though, it became clear to me that they were violating their bodies' instinctive
wisdom and overriding it with what seemed to them to be superior wisdom,
the teachings associated with meditation.

Whenever this happens, when we have been denying ourselves and then in meditation we temporarily become whole, it is usually painful and terrifying to some extent.

In each case it is remarkable how instantly the healing started. Phyllis had several minutes of sacred-feeling peacefulness, and then she started into the healing of memories,

where her deepest pain came to the surface to be felt and transformed. Jane meditated very deeply from the first few minutes, and she had no problem during sessions with me, but when meditating at home she ran into the sleep issue the very first day.

I have always found that it is much better, in the long run, to have the wounds be cleansed, even if it hurts. It is uncomfortable to sit there and feel this process, but afterward what a relief. But there was nothing in the PR blitz surrounding meditation that prepared Steve, Phyllis, or Jane for what meditation actually felt like. There was no explicit promise of healing that would lure them beyond their initial pain.

They were aware of the benefits of meditation, as reported by medical researchers. It sounded like a sensible thing to do. But right away they each in their own way had to deal with what is called unstressing—meaning the gyrations the body goes through to let go of the chronic stress that is choking off the flow of life.

During the early 1970s I never described in my introductory sessions how much meditation could hurt, how intense the pain could be when you dive down and face your deepest, most shattering fears. I myself had been through incredible pain in meditation, in the year I spent in a room meditating and doing yoga all day as part of my teacher training. But it has been so totally healed that I forgot the pain and remembered only the healing.

All this shows that any and all approaches to meditation have their flaws. Every school, no matter how enlightened some of the teachers may be, is severely limited—it is appropriate for maybe 1 percent or less of any given population in the Western world. No one approach to meditation is universal. Teachers are in general only good at teaching people who are very much like themselves. They are also only good when they have the courage to let the student be better than them, and in my experience my students are usually better than me at all sorts of things. I learn startling new things about meditation every single day, it seems, and every person I work with one-to-one comes up with interesting and fresh solutions. I often just create a situation in which the student can have an insight, and then I learn from it also.

During the time I was conducting my Ph.D. research, between 1978 and 1985, I sought out meditators of all stripes to interview about their experiences—everyone from Christian monks to Sikhs. I was amazed at how many self-taught meditators I met, people who just made up their own meditation and did it happily and consistently for years.

I have never been able to tell in advance how far a person will go in terms of accepting the uncomfortable aspects of meditation. For that reason I suspect that it is not a matter of "kind of person" or typology. It is a decision a person makes to trust his or her own healing process as it occurs when he or she lets go. Whether we make that decision in each moment depends upon all of who we are and what we have learned from love and life. It takes courage to recognize meditation as a time when you can release control utterly and allow the natural wisdom of your body to take over and heal you.

If you and I were sitting together, one on one, as you explored meditation, you wouldn't need to know all of this. We would just begin, and then as obstacles came up we would deal with them. If any kind of inner obstacle came up during the session, we would within seconds stop meditating, open our eyes, and talk about it until you had the information you needed to continue. In that way, you would not develop any bad habits, and you would have a good chance of getting into a fulfilling, healthy meditation habit. You would learn to handle whatever your inner life was tossing at you each moment. Mostly we would explore what you really love, and construct your meditation practice to be like that. This helps you to be at home in meditation right away, which makes the meditation deeper and more powerful.

This is why it is worthwhile to read through all of this discussion of experiences, slowly, over a period of weeks before beginning meditation. Again, the meditation part is simple; it's your incredible life that is so intricate and needs to be handled with joy and respect. You will be much better off if you begin that way, from the very first few seconds.

Ultimately, whether you meditate only once or you get into the habit of meditating every day, each and every meditation is an intimate journey of discovery that changes moment by moment as you travel through your inner life. The only way you can handle it is one breath at a time, breath after breath.

The Rest/Activation Cycle in Meditation

So now that you know all that meditation should be, what exactly should it be like? First off, during meditation you will find yourself fluctuating between restfulness and restlessness. The cycle may take only 15 seconds, in which you settle in, feel at ease, and then start thinking of things to do. Or it may take 3 minutes, or 5 minutes, or longer. Even when we feel mainly restful for a prolonged period of time, say 10 or 20 minutes, this long rhythm will be made up of many shorter fluctuations. It is only very occasionally that a sense of total stillness dawns and lasts more than a few seconds.

Movement toward restfulness. Toward resting in the self.

Movement toward action. Expressing the self in the world.

These two cycle again and again. Going inward to bathe in the self, then orienting to the outer world and readying to manifest your essence in living.

You never know what your cycles will look like or feel like in a given meditation. You might be exhausted after a long, busy day doing a million things and be surprised to find that when you sit down and meditate you feel pure pleasure—ecstatic even. Other times you may feel great when you start meditating and then you fall asleep and dream the whole time. Be willing to be surprised.

You should expect that at least half of your meditating time will feel like you are just thinking, sorting through sensations, conversations, actions, and impressions. This is healthy and good. In fact, one of the greatest things you can do for your meditation is to make peace with this cycle. Welcome thoughts in meditation. Otherwise you will condemn yourself to an eternal struggle.

Take a few conscious breaths, close your eyes, and watch the flow of thoughts. Notice the way your cycle appears just now.

If you start paying attention to your body, you will notice that during the day your bodily energies fluctuate. Sometimes you are more energetic and sometimes

WHAT MEDITATION FEELS LIKE

Nodding off	Sitting on the beach
Lots and lots of thoughts	Getting a massage
Daydreaming	Sleeping
An incredible rest	Feeding on the silence
Recharging	Total repose
Riding waves of excitement	Electricity
Worrying	Constant change

As you can see, these are all manifestations of the body's instinctive sensibility. The body moves from one tone to another in response to your needs. Often, the experience changes every few seconds.

more restful. Your body by nature follows something like a 90-minute to 2-hour cycle, where you will feel more energetic for most of that time and then for about 20 minutes you will crave to take a break. (This is why union rules allow for rest breaks or coffee breaks several times during the day.) These cycles are called ultradian rhythms. Attuning to your ultradian rhythms will help you ride the rest/activation cycles within meditation.

About half the time when you are meditating, you will be experiencing the play of opposites in terms of relaxation/tension. There is a lively interaction between deep relaxation and the need your body has to release chronically constricted emotional/muscular tensions. We all tend to hold different muscles on guard against feeling—either because we anticipate attack or criticism, or because we have voices in our heads that criticize us, or because we are striving to do our best. If you have a sense of hurrying, or that your natural pace is not fast enough, you will tend to chronically tighten your muscles in some way, somewhere—the neck, the shoulders, the stomach, the pelvis. These may be areas of your body that chronically ache, or where you have health problems.

In meditation your body will relax, and then you will think of the things that make you tense, and then feel the panic or discomfort underneath the tension— and if you stay there, the fear will tend to be washed out of your body. This process sounds very uncomfortable, and it sometimes is. But because you are sitting on your sofa breathing easily, in a kind of conscious rest that's deeper than sleep, it is usually more like watching a movie in a theater—maybe one that has vibrating seats.

You can learn to experience this flow of life as a rich current of something like electricity. It's nice to know that some thoughts have nothing to do with stress; rather, they can be classified as excitement. You are rarin' to go. You experience contact with some inner level of your being and you want to go out into the world and share it. When you go inside, you get excited about opening up this part of yourself you have discovered and relating it to the world.

So what does meditation feel like? Well, what does the deepest and best rest you have ever had feel like? Meditation is the laziest thing you can do, ever. It feels as intimate as your favorite music—rhythm, vibrations, tinglings, electricity, massage, feeding on the silence. It feels as intimate as sex—or more so.

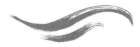

The Essential Rhythm of Meditative Experience

You are going about your business. Maybe it is early morning and you have a busy day ahead of you and you want to be at your best. Or it is the end of the day and you want to recover. Or maybe you are hurting in some way, or recovering from some hurt. You sense that some elixir is needed to restore balance. You feel the call to do something to take care of yourself. You are being beckoned, invited within.

You refuse to go. *I don't have time. . . . This isn't the place. . . . Maybe later I'll learn to meditate. . . .*

The call gets stronger. More insistent.

Finally, you take some time to be with yourself. Perhaps some instinctive knowledge of meditation comes to you and you start to settle in.

You close your eyes and approach the threshold. One of the threshold guardians attacks you with thoughts or sensations: *There are things to do! Places to go! You don't have the discipline to meditate, fool!*

You face these thoughts, let them flow through you, and you remain. You cultivate an interest in your breathing, your mantra, a bodily sensation, a part of your body that calls you. You find some inner allies—sensations or perceptions that lead you deeper into yourself.

Enemies appear in the form of fears and other feelings you want to turn away from. You suddenly feel as if you have to abandon meditation and run away, do anything—clean out the closets, scrub the floor, watch TV—*do* anything but face this. Some thought about work attacks you—an image of somebody you hate or fear, a bodily feeling that you do not want to admit to, an impulse you don't like in yourself. Because you are relaxed and have let your guard down, it comes at you. It is ac-

THE RHYTHM OF MEDITATIVE EXPERIENCE

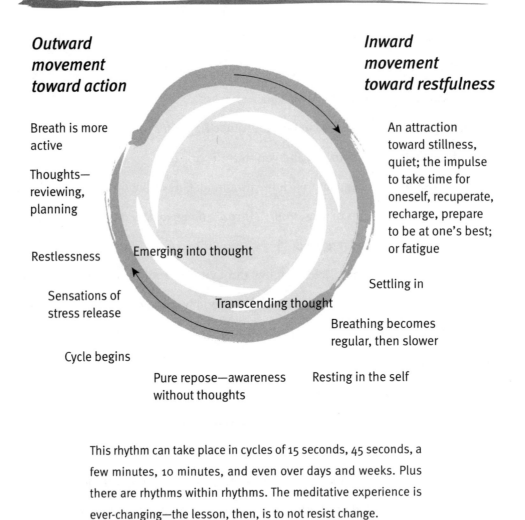

Outward movement toward action

Breath is more active

Thoughts—reviewing, planning

Restlessness

Sensations of stress release

Cycle begins

Emerging into thought

Transcending thought

Pure repose—awareness without thoughts

Inward movement toward restfulness

An attraction toward stillness, quiet; the impulse to take time for oneself, recuperate, recharge, prepare to be at one's best; or fatigue

Settling in

Breathing becomes regular, then slower

Resting in the self

This rhythm can take place in cycles of 15 seconds, 45 seconds, a few minutes, 10 minutes, and even over days and weeks. Plus there are rhythms within rhythms. The meditative experience is ever-changing—the lesson, then, is to not resist change.

tually already there in your body, but by keeping busy you have managed to push it away. Now you are too relaxed to maintain the inner wall against yourself. *Arrrrrrrgggggghhhhh.* Hand-to-hand combat with the enemy ensues.

You are killed; or you kill the enemy and eat his liver; or the enemy turns into a beautiful woman, an angel, God, or a magical power—an ally. In any case, you stay there, inside, and the fear melts away. *Ahhh.* You settle into yourself some more. You really let go. Minutes pass in enjoyment.

Ahhhhhhhhhhhhhhhhhhhhhhhhhhhhhhhhh . . .

Energy is liberated from your denial mechanisms and gushes through your body. An elixir permeates your cells. What a sublime feeling. *I am healed. I am finally myself.* You have contact with the divine, or with the life force, or with the postorgasmic state of total silence.

You are aware of nothing, no time passes, you are merged with the universe for a split second or more. You have a moment of pure being. The world is the same, but you are changed. Your body is suffused with wisdom and peace.

Then thoughts come. At first you are not aware that thoughts have come. You are just really involved in planning that party, thinking about your car, musing about the garage and how you really should clean it out, thinking about sex, thinking about the friends you haven't seen or the movies you haven't seen. Then you become aware that you are thinking. *Oh no, I blew it! I was really peaceful and then I ruined it by thinking!*

Looking Good

One of my favorite effects of meditation is the way my sense of vision is enhanced after a sitting. My eyes seem to drink in the colors and radiance of the world. A vividness and internal luminosity permeate the environment and delight my eyes. People look much better to me. Even after more than 30 years, my vision continues to be refreshed by meditation.

Damn! Then an ally reminds you, like Obi-Wan Kenobi talking to Luke Skywalker, *Thoughts are part of meditation,* and you settle into peacefulness again.

Then it's *Uh-oh, gotta go! What time is it? How long have I been sitting here? What day is it? I have to go make breakfast/dinner/a report/the commute/an appointment.* Then again, you suddenly become aware that your mind has been wandering. All that urgency is just a feeling of tension underlying your thinking. But it actually *is* getting on time to finish meditating. So you let go and just sit there—and sink even deeper than before.

Now, suddenly, you don't want to get up. It's like not wanting to wake up in the morning. *Oh, just a few more minutes. . . .* You move your hands a little—*My God, where are my hands? I am so relaxed I can hardly move!*—and you open your eyes a little, but they close by themselves. *Ohhhhh, just give me a minute. . . .*

This is sort of what happens during meditation every 20 minutes or so. There are innumerable variations, of course, but listening to people report on their experiences over the years, I keep hearing some version of this again and again. The major characters tend to appear as bodily sensations and as verbal thoughts more than as images. They do not seem exotic, as in movies and epics, but have their power because they are so familiar.

This is the rhythm of meditative experience. Get used to it.

The Whole Body Scan

The basic teaching of the body scan has been around forever. The purpose of paying attention to a particular body part or area is to enrich your sensory awareness of that part and at the same time to access its healing power for use by the whole of your body. As you develop sensory awareness, you have more and more interesting details to pay attention to, which makes your overall sense of self richer and more textured and your healing instincts more responsive.

When you place your attention in any body part, no matter how often you do it, you enter a known but always-new landscape. The body scan technique I'm suggesting is not about tossing a modicum of attention at a place in your body and then trying

4

QUESTIONING THE BODY

As you move through the body scan explorations in this chapter, ask yourself the following questions. Some of these questions—and their answers—you will immediately understand, some will make sense to you soon, and others may not come to your senses for years.

- What does the pained part want?
- What sensations can you detect there?
- How does the part feel—hot, cold, strong, weak?
- How does the circulation of energy flow?
- What movement possibilities are there?
- What kind of numbness or blankness do you feel there?
- What sorts of electricity do you feel?
- What senses help you to notice the part?
- What is the best feeling you have ever had in this body part?
- What is the worst?
- What emotion is held in this body part?
- What instinctive quality is related to this body part?
- When do you become aware of this part of your body in the course of a day?

You might also explore the following senses as they relate to the body part that's calling:

- Envisioning
- Motion
- Touching
- Balance
- Vibrating with sound
- Joint sensing

to control it or whip it into shape. It is about attending to your whole self with curiosity, tenderness, and love. This concept may seem complicated or confusing at this point, but you will get the feel for it as you explore. Basically, the idea of the body scan is to get quiet and find where your attention is being called in your body.

Sometimes when you are doing a body scan, your attention will be called to an area not because there is pain but just because it is interesting for awareness to rest there in the legs or the pelvis or the heart. You are inhabiting yourself. You are cultivating your kinesthesia—the aesthetic sense of pleasure in the body—so that when you are paying attention in general to the body, doing a body scan, or dealing with pain in a particular part of the body, you have a richer sensory palate to work with.

Developing your kinesthetic sense is analogous to fully appreciating a band, symphony, or choral performance. You can listen to the overall effect and enjoy it, and then at some point you might find yourself separating out each individual element: this voice, those words, that instrument. Awareness of the parts helps you return to the sense of the whole gestalt of the music with a greater sense of enjoyment. In the same way, when you are suffering from pain in the body or soul, you can access the pleasure and peacefulness you have developed in the different parts of your body to help deal with the discomfort.

The purpose of the body scan is to promote full circulation throughout your whole being. Sometimes a body part calls for more energy, as when it's cold or hungry. Another part or place in the body may have an excess of energy (too hot), congestion, or compression that needs to be released into the body—the life force has gotten trapped and needs to be freed up. By attending to the individual body parts that call your attention, the balance in your whole system can readily be restored. In becoming sensitive to all these nuances of what is being asked for, you are training your attention to be healing attention.

Here are some of the body parts and the roles that they play.

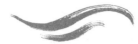

Embracers—The Hands and Arms

The hands have healing power. You may or may not have ever explored this, so we will begin now. The hands are symbolic of attention, and when you are feeling yourself internally in meditation, it is as if you are touching yourself inside with invisible hands. By starting with the hands, you are invoking your own healing power, which you can carry to the other body parts.

With the arms we can embrace and draw close what we love, and we can gather into ourselves. The arms are channels of energy that come right from the heart center and express through the hands. We can also push away when we need to—anything we no longer want or don't want to deal with at the moment. The ability to push off, fend off, and send someone or some emotion or problem packing is crucial for emotional and physical health.

THE WHOLE BODY SCAN MAP

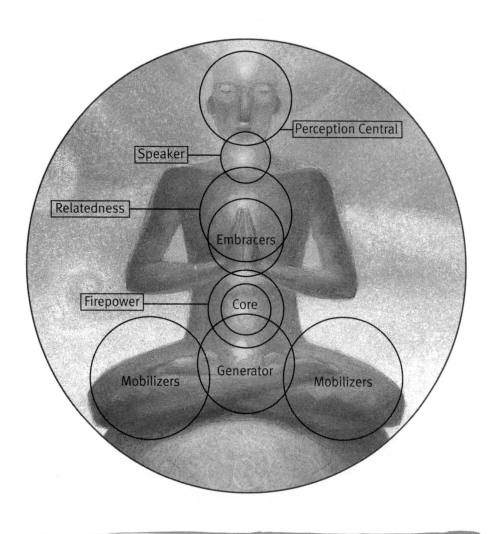

The hands and arms taken together are the expression of the heart. They connect us to the world. We touch ourselves, then we reach out and touch others.

To explore the hands and arms, spend a few moments doing each of the following activities in an unhurried manner.

Hand it to your hands: Look at your hands. Touch them with each other. Thank them for their capacity, for their ability to touch, to give and receive. Rub them together, then put your palms over your eyes and feel the warmth.

Appreciate all the things the hands can do—look down at your hands and explore moving one or both of them in all manner of intricate little movements. Feel the strength in the hands and arms, and yet recall how tenderly they can touch and sense and embrace. Run through the list of the instincts in your mind and appreciate how the hands have a hand in exploring, grooming, hunting, gathering, and participating in the other motions of life.

Wrap one hand up in the other and simply feel the warmth. Do this for a minute or so. Then pause to feel the energy circulating in your hands. If you like, imagine that the life force is streaming out of every finger.

Magnetic hands: Sit or stand with your palms pointing in toward each other, about a foot apart. Feel the magnetism, the attraction between the palms. Play with the distance—farther apart, closer together. Each bit of distance has its joy: Sometimes when the hands are farther away, they can feel each other more; sometimes you want to move them closer. Celebrate how your hands can sense the magnetism.

Blessing hands: Slowly bring your hands together, to touch each other. Then run your hands over the entire area of the skin, everywhere your hands can reach. Reach your hands into the space in front of you and gather in any element you want or crave or feel you need: healing waters, sacred fire, the perfect vibration, the right healing magnetism. Let your hands be drenched with that element, made out of it, conduits for it. Then bring your hands in to touch any part of your body that needs it.

Claim your space: Gesture with your arms to indicate your boundary. Wave your hands around in a ceremonial fashion to claim the space. Spread your energies, as if you are establishing a perimeter and your place within it. Take a few breaths and notice whatever bodily sensations you feel. Now raise the arms above the head and reach upward. This space is yours too.

Reach into the area in front of your torso. Tilt your hands in different ways and note the difference. The palms facing outward is the universal STOP sign. The palms facing in toward your body is a chi gung, or movement meditation—a position of gathering energy into yourself.

Reach out to both sides, and even behind you. Know that this space is yours for now.

Secret longing: What secret longing do your hands hold? Do you want to touch or be touched in a certain way? Whatever that secret is, you do not have to tell anyone, but welcome it into the space of your meditation.

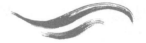

Mobilizers—The Feet and Legs

The feet are the parts of you that touch the earth when you walk and connect you to the ground. The feet are small and take up little space and yet they support the entire weight of the body. It is nothing short of miraculous how this system of little bones and tendons that are your feet can be so powerful and durable.

The legs have an upper part, the thigh, and a lower part, the calves and shin, connected by the knee. With this deceptively simple structure you have an amazing range of mobility. The legs are your mobilizers. You can walk, run, jump, kick, swim, twine around a loved one, and stand. You can move toward what you want or flee from what you do not want.

There is a great stability to the legs. They connect you to the ground, the foundation. Although mobile, the legs and feet are like the trunk of a tree, and beneath your feet are energetic roots connecting you to the depths of the Earth. The stability comes from the continual sensing of your relationship to the ground. When you walk, your feet sense variations in the surface below you and automatically adjust.

The legs and feet are extensions of the root center, located between the legs in the area of the perineum. This is a magical spot, cherished by both lovers and meditators, for here primal earth energy mixes with the human realm of feeling. Perineal energy is not sexual, it is the primal, earthy joy to be alive. It is a springing up from the earth in irresistible force.

Planted firmly on the ground: Stand and feel your relationship to the ground, how your legs are carrying you. Stand and breathe with an awareness of the earth below you. With each inbreath, energy flows up from the earth to support you. With each breath out, the used energy flows back into the earth. Now shift your weight from one foot to the other, slowly. Feel how immediate your sense of balance is, how your entire body is alert to gravity and continually orienting toward it.

Sit in a chair with your feet on the ground. Feel your feet and legs connected to the earth. This is one of my favorites. Although I am comfortable sitting cross-legged for many hours at a time, I often prefer to sit with my feet on the ground. It's a great posture, and much better for your knees.

Moving in the world: A stroll or a meander can be a moving meditation when you pay attention to all your senses as you glide along. Feel the power of your legs as you walk. Pay attention to your feet as they touch the ground. What quality does that meeting have? What is your natural rhythm of walking? Find it, be with for a while, and then vary it. Move faster, then slower. Then slower still. Be aware of the new information coming up through your legs and feet. See how slowly you can walk and still enjoy yourself.

Notice your breath rhythm and how it might change as your gait changes. Be aware of and grateful for the part your legs play in all the instinctive motions of life, exploring, playing, and loving.

Walk as if you are going to meet your lover.

Walk as if you are with your lover on the way to somewhere and you are dawdling, trying to stretch out the moment.

Walk as if you are on a hunt.

Walk quietly, as if you are stalking something.

Walk as if God is in every step.

187

Walk as if you were walking toward a meeting with God.

Walk with the awareness of walking in the universe—you are on a tiny sphere of a planet, out on the edge of one galaxy out of many.

Once you get the feel for walking with these tones, you can shift between them in a fraction of a second. Anytime you walk anywhere, you can play with an instinctive tone for a moment here and there.

Breath meditation with the feet and legs: Lie on your back and prop your feet up, maybe on a couch. Breathe and imagine that your feet and legs are very buoyant. By doing this you are reversing the circulation of blood in the area. This is good for relieving tension in the legs.

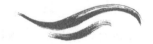

Perception Central—The Head

The head is quite a package. It contains the eyes, the ears, the inner ears, the nose, the mouth, the tongue, and the brain. The brain itself is made up of many parts and layers, all of which process different kinds of information and somehow talk to one another.

Breath flows in and out from the head, through the nostrils and mouth. We take in food through an opening in the front of the head, and break the food down in a process called chewing. Whew! What a lot of sensing, sensory information processing, and substance handling.

Ask yourself, *Where is my "I," my center of awareness?* For many of us in the modern world, the head is the center of our sense of self. People living closer to nature sometimes point to their bellies or hearts as the center of awareness. Martial artists and dancers might point to their lower bellies.

It is very easy for us moderns to have congested energy in the head because we are thinking so much, dealing with information overload, too much responsibility, too many things to track. During meditation, one of the challenges is how to deal with all the thoughts flying everywhere. You need to learn to immediately give your brain what it needs.

Lighten up: The antidote to too many thoughts is a softening, a letting go. For example, meditate on the feeling of your brain floating like a cloud in the sky. Soften your face, your eyes, your mouth, your cheeks, your lips. Imagine a flow of energy down from your head to your feet and to the ground. Give yourself space above the head and around the head.

Notice your inner theater: Catch yourself visualizing or seeing a mental image sometime, or create the experience now. Think of a picture of anything and notice where your mental screen is. Is it in front of you, down slightly, or up? Are there several screens? Do you have picture-in-picture, like some television sets? Can you make your screen larger, panoramic, IMAX, or 3-D? Form a mental image, any image you enjoy, and breathe with it. Let the dimensionality and flow of breath support your image creation. Give yourself more subjective space within which to think. You may have formed the habit as a child of being hunched over a desk, crowding your thoughts. Give yourself the whole universe to think in.

Breathe into the palate: Breathe in and out through your mouth for a few minutes; let the cooling air glide over the top of your tongue and touch the roof of your mouth. Let the breath blow through your thinking areas. It may feel as if the magnetism in the breath flows right up through the roof of the mouth into the base of the brain, soothing and bringing harmony.

LORIN'S NOTEBOOK

ROB: EYES SHUT, MOUTH OPEN

"I found that it helps immensely if I just sit and focus on letting go of all the muscles in and around the eye. Of course, there are many layers to this. Eventually one will be able to let go of the eyes and have all the muscles in and around the eyes completely relaxed, absolutely nothing going on. If the old programming comes in and wants to tense up the eyes, just bring the focus back and let go of control.

"Once this is done, you will find that the whole body relaxes when the eyes are completely relaxed. Even extremely tense shoulder muscles will go limp. The face will go limp. This is a very relaxed state for the body.

"Next, if one can learn to hang out in this completely relaxed eye state, various parts of the body—especially the eyes, face, neck, shoulders—may and probably will want to move around on their own. It's a bit of a paradox. The eyes are totally relaxed, the meditator is letting go of control of all the muscles, and yet many muscles will move on their own in this way or that. This movement is another stress valve being opened, allowing the memories or trauma

Slow motion of the head: Let the back of your neck be mobile, and make some invisible motions with your head. Feel where "up" is and then move your head in a tiny circle, about an inch in diameter, slowly around that spot where up is. Then let the circle and the motion become smaller.

to slowly disappear from the muscles and the muscles to do their own thing. When you have mastered this technique, you can quickly relax your body in any situation—even in public."

Another one of Rob's favorite techniques is yawning. You simply make yourself yawn a few times, stretching the jaws, and then give the reflex a chance to take over.

"This really helps me decrease stress at a maximum rate, and it's especially useful when driving.

"The mouth is opened and the tongue moves around it—inside and way outside, in such a fashion that the tongue movement eventually produces a major yawn. After the first yawn, the tongue movement is done again, with the mouth open and also moving until a second yawn is produced. And so on. After 10 to 20 yawns, stress is dramatically decreased. True, the more yawns done, the harder it is usually to get another one out, but the later ones tend to clear stress even more. Yawning is especially good for reducing adrenaline-rush stress that affects all of the body but is harbored in the abdominal region."

Hands to head: Place the palms of your hands on the top of your head, fingers almost touching, your hands just barely touching the hair on your head. Slowly lift your hands upward, noting the sensations. In synchronization with your breathing, gently pulsate your hands up and down a mere fraction of an inch. Explore motions such as this to see if you find pleasure and interest. This may help you cultivate the sense of having more space to think in.

Vibrate the head with sound: Play with humming and chanting any sounds. Check out what you feel when you close your mouth and make a *Mmmm* sound. Hum in such a way that your throat, cheeks, tongue, and anywhere else in your head you can get to is vibrated. Hum the first sound that comes to you.

Take a deep breath and hum a longer duration: *Mmmmmmmmmmmmmm . . .* or whatever sound you chose. Feel it come out through your face. Release the sound through your face. There are resonant chambers in the front of your skull in the area of the face, called sinuses, and they receive the sound and amplify it. Make the sound high and then low. Where does the sound go? Where does the vibration move to? Continue to take deep breaths and exhale with a sound. Vary the sound. Now issue a sound that makes your lips buzz.

You can do this exercise for any length of time you like. On a practical level, you might find that 3 minutes at the beginning of meditation helps your practice.

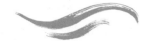

Relatedness—The Chest

The chest is where the heart and lungs do their magic of combining the breath of life with the blood of life and sending it everywhere in the body. This alchemy of transmutation goes on night and day, whether we are awake or asleep, as long as we live. Think about how many times a day your heart beats, how many breaths your lungs process—do the math.

There is a spiritual heart in the vicinity of the physical heart and it is also about giving and receiving certain kinds of energy. It processes energy in motion, called emotion. Whenever we are in a feeling relationship to anything or anyone, there are many movements in our hearts. We can feel as if there are vibrating chords of energies streaming, pulsing, and humming with a musical harmony or disharmony.

In yoga, this heart center is called anahata, which means the unstruck chord, because its music has no beginning and no end. It hums on and on in a melody that can be heard as a symphony of silence or sound. All mantras are meant to remind you of the anahata, the resonance of your own heart. In meditation, you can appreciate the counterpoint rhythm of your heart and the heart of the universe.

Cherish your heartbeat: At different times of day, depending on how quiet you get, you may be able to feel your pulse in your arms, torso, or chest area. Take several deep breaths, and exhale fully. Find a rhythm to the breath that appeals to you in the moment. Continue to emphasize the exhale until you have done about seven breaths this way.

Then emphasize the inbreath for seven breaths. That means you give more attention to it, and a little bit of oomph.

Now close your eyes and breathe in an easy, smooth rhythm and feel around in your chest for your heartbeat. After a minute, if you don't feel it, place the fingers of one of your hands on the opposing wrist and feel your pulse there. Simply give thanks for the steady, faithful beating of the heart.

Joy to the world: One way to pay attention to the heart as a feeling center is to remember what you love. Think of those people, animals, and places that make your heart glad. This technique seems very prosaic, the mental equivalent of those photographs people have on their desks, the kids and grandparents. In fact, that is its power—it's just like what we do anyway when we are happy. In this simple way, bring up the happiest feelings you know, the experience of joy when you feel grateful to the world for the gift of life.

Now pay attention to the sensations in the chest area, the sense of motion or ache, or of lightness and flow. Breathe with those sensations, support them, encourage them, bless them with your breath. With your awareness, be sensitive to the entire area from the sternum, the chest bone, to the spine. Notice the different textures of sensation in each part of the upper torso.

Admire your heart for having the courage to feel. With the rhythm of the breath, support the faster rhythm of the pulse.

Listening with the heart: Put on the greatest music you know and listen from the heart. It could be Bach, choral, jazz—anything you really, truly love that makes you feel good. Lying down or sitting, listen to the music with your whole being and then find your way in so that you are listening from your heart. This will make sense as you get into it. Practice this for a few months. It is a great talent. Some day you may save a relationship by being able to listen from the heart to someone you love.

Secret longing: Let your arms move in gestures of receiving and giving. Do these gestures quickly and then more slowly. Then more slowly still. Then more slowly than you have ever moved. Feel the emotional richness of this movement as you say something like, *I feel in my heart my connectedness to everything I love.*

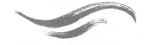

Firepower—The Solar Plexus

Located at the base of the ribs is the powerful muscle of the diaphragm. The diaphragm is a pump that pulls breath into your lungs and flushes it back out many times a minute. This is the breath that feeds the fires of life. From ancient times this area has been perceived as an important body center related to the sun. The area is even called the solar plexus to indicate its relationship to the sun's radiant power. Located here are the organs of digestion that allow us to take the raw material of food and transform it, so that the body can turn it into energy, movement, and expression.

When we feel crowded or threatened, a lot happens in the solar plexus: Breathing is often constricted, the adrenals are activated, digestion stops. By freeing up your breathing, you can learn to keep the tension from congesting your solar plexus as you move through your day. You can exit from false feeling of emergency very quickly and save a lot of energy and frustration.

Diaphragmatic breathing: Lie on the ground on your back. Perhaps put a little pillow under your head and another under your knees. Rest in this way for several breaths. Bring your hands to the area above your navel and just below your ribs. Place your fingertips at your midline and notice the motions underneath your hands. As you inhale, your lower ribs and belly expand outward. As you exhale, they soften and your hands sink in slightly.

Enjoy this movement, exploring the full range of your breath. Experiment with longer inhales and exhales.

Now play with taking a deep breath. Hold it at the top of the inhalation and feel the stretch of your breathing muscles, ribs, and skin. When you exhale and release the stretch there is often a surge of pleasure.

I know many very experienced meditators who do this as their main practice each day. They just lie down, place their hands on their bellies, and feel their breathing for half an hour twice a day; this tunes them up. These are some of the happiest, busiest, healthiest meditators I know, so I have interviewed them. What I find is that as they lie there simply breathing, they let the instinctive tone be whatever it wants to be. They let themselves orbit between resting, being massaged by breath, sleeping and dreaming, feeding on the air, tenderly touching with inner awareness all the areas of the body that seem to call for it, listening to the hum of energy in the body, and letting their attention even out the flow of energies so that everything everywhere feels well-tuned. What they do is basically give themselves a head-to-toe massage and healing treatment every day.

Pulsing breath: Sit upright and exhale in little bursts of breath through the mouth, lips gently pursed, and make a *hu* sound as you exhale. Continue in this way for several minutes.

This is similar in effect to the breath of fire exercise beloved by many different yoga traditions, in that it increases circulation to the diaphragm. Imagine that you are stoking the fires of life within your body. Just do a little bit of this at a time until you get used to the feeling. Even one minute can be intense at first. This exploration is a celebration of breath and a way to develop awareness of your diaphragm.

When you get tired of the *hu* breath, just sit there and enjoy the streaming sensations.

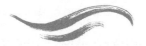

Generator—The Pelvis and Lower Belly

The lower belly is the center of gravity of the body, and the center of movement. It is also, delightfully, the area where the sexual organs are, with all their amazing nerve endings and possibilities of sensation. By being centered in the lower abdomen, dancers, martial artists, and gymnasts are free to gyrate in every possible direction and still stay oriented to gravity.

There is deep feeling in the lower belly. Often the most difficult emotions, the most intolerable grief and rage, get buried here. In order to hold these feelings back, deep muscles have to tighten and stay chronically tensed. Over time, this tensing can restrict blood flow to the organs and even cause lower back pain. When these emotions are released, people may shake, sob, or scream from the belly. A truly deep laugh is called a belly laugh. The Japanese say, "He has belly," meaning gravitas. Let yourself have belly.

The sexual organs are located in the pelvis, of course, an area of great feeling. If we feel safe to inhabit our sexuality, we may experience currents of electricity, joy, and creative energy flowing through our bodies almost continuously. These energies constantly modulate themselves, changing in tone and pitch, stimulating the rest of the body with the zest for life. If we do not feel safe enough to relax into our natural, healthy sexuality, the whole body is deprived of this vital force. This has nothing to do with acting out sexual impulses. It's about letting our energies flow freely without stifling them.

Rock your pelvis: Sit in a chair with your feet on the ground. Let your spine be free to move around. Feel how your pelvis rests on the chair—there are sensations of contact—and let your weight pull you down into the chair. As you explore this, notice how the chair is holding you up. This is an extremely simple observation.

Gently begin to rock forward and back and side to side. You will feel the weight shift in your lower back, hipbones, sacrum, and tailbone. After exploring for a few seconds or a few days, you will develop the ability to sense many different areas.

Belly breath: Sit in a chair and place your hands, fingertips touching, below the belly button. Notice whatever movement you feel as you breathe. Rest in that way for seven breaths. Then begin doing long and slow exhalations, emptying the breath out completely. With your fingertips, feel those wonderful muscles working. Do seven long exhalation breaths, then sit back and notice how you feel.

Be aware of the flow of breath and invite yourself to experience the breath in a continuous flow of feeling from your nose all the way down to your lower belly. The air does not actually flow down into the lower belly, but the sensation of breath permeates into the pelvis because the lower abdominal muscles are involved in breathing. This is a joyous feeling, a sense of wholeness. If this is unfamiliar to you, just become interested in the lower belly. Gradually, your attention will find sources of pleasure there to be with and you will learn more and more about the full-body breath.

The belly relaxes more when you are lying down, so after doing this sitting up once or twice, explore this in a supine position. Lie on your back with a pillow under your knees and go through the same process.

Ho-ho-ho: Chant "Ho-ho-ho" in brief bursts. Contract the belly with each "Ho." Do this for 1 minute, then breathe normally and notice your sensa-

SELF-STRANGULATION

When you tell yourself that you can't handle an emotion that arises, you place a difficult burden on the body. The nervous system and muscles will try to protect you by partly strangling the body part involved in the emotion. They will keep on doing this until you give orders to do otherwise.

tions. Do another eight "Ho's", then pause for eight counts, then breathe another eight "Ho's". Do five cycles of this.

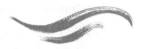

Core—The Spine

The spine is at the very core of your body. It is the primary support structure for the upper body. All the other bones and muscles hang on the spine. Inside of the spine is the spinal cord, which carries information between your brain and the nerves throughout your body. There is also a channel for cerebrospinal fluid, which is pumped through the core of the spine and feeds the brain. In subtle states of awareness you can feel a tiny pulse of this fluid as it circulates through the brain and into the cavity of the spinal cord. The ancient yogis felt this fluid and called it nectar, one of the great elixirs of meditation.

Keeping the spine fluid is a key to your health. When areas of the spine become compressed, which can happen easily when you do not move enough during daily life, it affects the whole body.

The lower spine, for example, is an area of pain for many people. The abdominal muscles help support the lower back, and keeping them toned can prevent a great deal of lower back pain. The spine takes the burdens of life you carry in more ways than just the physical. If there is a feeling you are afraid of, a rage that you do not want to consciously own up to, you may inadvertently wind up dumping it on your lower back or neck or other part of your spine. Many people have found that when they acknowledge their rage or fear, they unburden the spine from the need to stay constricted, and their back pain disappears.

Keeping the spine supple is a major way of slowing the aging process. To have a supple spine may make you feel like a kid. The curves of the spine allow it to move in an undular fashion that absorbs shock. This wavelike motion is often compared to the serpentine movement of a snake.

The symbol of the medical profession is the caduceus, two snakes twining around a staff, which represents the flow of life energy through the spine. At the top of the staff is a sphere, which represents the brain, and wings, representing enlightenment. This is actually a profound meditation symbol, and you can imagine your own body merging with the image. Doing so is a suggestion, an encouragement to your life energies to flow freely and in balance. There is great motion in the image, and great stillness.

Caduceus meditation: Sit upright on a chair with your feet on the ground. Begin to sway gently, letting your spine curve in different directions: forward and back, side to side, and at every angle of the compass. Let your range of motion be multidimensional. Play with the motion, explore, find what is soothing, enjoy the massage of it.

Feel the movement rippling through your spine, all the way from your tailbone to the base of your neck. Let your head bobble with the gentle wave motions, just riding on top.

If you'd like, you can visualize the two snakes undulating. Imagine that they are actually making love, eternally playing with the polarities of male and female, yin and yang, in and out, up and down.

This is an extremely simple exercise once you get used to it. The motion can just take over and continue spontaneously if you want it to, as if you were listening to music and swaying. At the end, sit still and sense the cerebrospinal fluid pulsing. Enjoy the tiny sensations, the afterglow of the movement.

You can do this for a few seconds anywhere and anytime you want a break, because it can be made to look just like a natural stretching movement. You'll see people wiggle their butts in their chairs every once in a while.

Lower back meditation: Lie on your back with your knees bent, feet flat on the floor. Take several breaths and feel the support of the ground. Simply notice your weight pressing into the ground.

Now become aware of the small of your back, the gentle curve of the lumbar spine and sacrum. As you inhale, increase that curve very slightly. Just arch your back almost imperceptibly. As you exhale, gently release the lower back toward the floor. Let the back of your waist and sacrum melt into the floor. Continue with this gentle undulation, arching as you inhale and melting as you exhale.

After you get used to this motion, which may take a few days, begin to be active on the exhale, freely rocking the sacrum forward and back. This exhaling movement also engages the deep abdominal muscles that support your lower back.

This should feel good, never painful. You are gently bringing movement to an area that often gets compressed and immobilized. One or two minutes is enough.

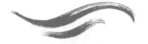

Speaker—The Neck and Throat

The neck is more than just the connection between the head and the rest of the body. The neck is a channel for breath, the home to the vocal cords, your built-in vibrational, musical, and communication apparatus.

The throat has to do with being heard, and to that extent is the seat of many control issues, because to live with other people we usually have to restrain our speech. But the throat also allows the rich experiences of your belly and heart to come out into expression. You can speak from the heart, speak from the belly, and speak from your whole body of experience. You can sing out what you are feeling inside, tell people you love them, share all your joys and sorrows.

Throat relaxer: Sit somewhere and let your chin drop a little, give your jaw permission to relax, and gently say to your tongue, *You can let go.* Then, on an exhalation, hear the sound of your breath flowing with a *hhhhhhh* sound. Make a soft, breathy sound, not vocalized, like a whisper. You are letting the air flow over your vocal cords without shaping them. That's it, do this for 1 to 3 minutes and enjoy how relaxing it is. We use our tongues and vocal cords so often, and rarely rest them.

Throat massage with sound: Actively sound out the vowels, such as *ahhhhhh*, in a way that pleasantly vibrates the throat. Do not strain; stay

LORIN'S NOTEBOOK

SARAH: HER HEART IN HER THROAT

One day I was reminded of the meaning of the phrase "My heart is in my throat." It happened in Santa Fe, New Mexico, where I used to live near the road to the opera. In the summer, singers would come to me for meditation coaching. In any given week the opera singers would see their voice coach and get a massage, so why not have some meditation coaching?

A 33-year-old English singer came for her first session, and then a week later she came back. When she walked in, she had a look about her that said she was about to break into tears, a look of great tenderness in her expression. I said, "You are so open, I can feel my heart vibrating in resonance with you."

Sarah told me this story. She had been to see her voice coach several days before, a 5-foot-tall English woman who coached many of the singers. Very fierce and demanding. The coach told her, "Listen, if you want to sing, you have to live with your throat open," and she showed her exercises for that.

Sarah cried and cried in the session. "But I can't function that way! I will cry all the time!"

"So cry all the time! Otherwise you will have no depth to your voice!"

Sarah said that for days she had been close to tears, and when she looked at

within your comfortable range. Play with *ahhhhhh* blending into *ohhhhhh*. At first say the sound out loud for a minute, then close your mouth and notice the changed vibrational sensations. Doing this for even a minute at the beginning of meditation can set a nice tone, and you may find over time that your voice becomes more relaxed.

certain people, like people in love and people with children, sometimes she did start crying.

Sarah grew up in a poor working-class family from an unfashionable suburb of London where women are drudges. She escaped by singing. By hardening herself, she made herself different from her mother. But now, if she was to open herself to her feelings, she had to grieve over the life she did not have, with a husband and children. The grief felt bottomless, the emotions so powerful.

Sarah and I did throat meditations, experiencing the hum of breath and sound in the throat, so that she would have a calming foundation underneath the tempestuous rising and falling of emotions—an inner stability.

With most people, the challenge is to get them to open up at all. But the voice coach did such a great job—better than I could have—that Sarah was open and ripe for incredible meditation experiences. Because she was so open to herself, and so attuned to sound, she had meditation experiences that would cause a yogi to be smitten with envy.

I said, "You sing songs that break people's hearts with beauty. Do you see that you have to be willing to have your heart broken open in order to sing?"

The heart breaks open, and you can die and be reborn many times a minute, with each heartbeat even.

Whole Body Dimensions

Beyond the body being the sum of its parts, there's a whole other range of dimensions or layers of the body that can enrich your experience when meditated upon. I find that paying attention to these dimensions surrounding and permeating the body for just a few seconds lights up my sense of being. Think the name of each and be aware of it for 10 seconds or so. Then take a breath and move on.

Skin — Skin is the interface between the inner and outer worlds, the membrane. An organ of absorption and elimination, it's the largest organ of the body. Skin is sensitive—it can feel warmth, touch as light as a feather. Are you sensitive to your environment? Emotional sensitivity can manifest itself as sensitive skin that's easily irritated.

Bones — Your skeleton is your support system, the inner structure that everything else hangs on. You want your bones to be strong but not brittle. The bones get strong from resisting gravity but will yield to the earth.

Immune system — The immune system identifies what is not a natural part of the body and eliminates it.

Circulation — Breathe into your whole body and imagine your entire body filling with breath. Other kinds of bodily circulation include blood (the life force) and lymph circulation.

Space—Let your entire body take up more space. Being in space is a transcendent feeling—the body as being part of something larger, the Earth, the stars.

Nervous system—The nerves are involved with sympathetic activation and parasympathetic restfulness. Your entire body is filigreed with these two systems of nerves.

When you are ready, try some of the following whole body explorations.

The Whole Body Salute: In this salutation, you move your hands and touch each body part appreciatively for a moment. What you are doing is saluting each part of your body, relating it to the whole, and letting your awareness dissolve into the whole.

Bring your fingertips together and touch your pubic bone, then the solar plexus, the heart, the throat, the forehead, and the top of the head, in that order. Continue the motion up above your head, reaching into space, then let your hands sweep out to the sides and down, back to the starting position, fingertips resting in your pubic area.

Do this three times.

Vary the speed at which you move. Linger for a breath in each spot. Then explore your preferences and move faster, move slower.

From there you can make up your own movement. Go for it. It is typical to feel awkward for 5 minutes when first doing this sort of exploration or when returning to it after an absence. Then, at some point, the poetry of the motion takes over and you find yourself spontaneously making up your own movements. It's a dance.

Do a dance: If at all possible, have some form of dance in your life on a regular basis. It could be anything, from hip-hop to ballroom, Latvian

Dance Sense

From dancers and divers to marathoners and mountaineers, professional and amateur athletes alike *know* that they must pay close attention to what their bodies have to tell them—or risk serious injury. Take for example the French dancer Sylvie Guillem, whom many consider to be the world's greatest ballerina. During an appearance with the Paris Opera Ballet, Ms. Guillem injured a muscle in her lower right leg. "It's the first time in my career that I have hurt myself in a performance," she told the *New York Times* in an article by Alan Riding (July 15, 2001). "I had a bad foot, but one is used to pain. I thought it was nothing and went on and began to compensate and then it came unstuck higher up. . . . If the body sends a message, you have to listen to it."

folk dancing to Afro-Brazilian macumba trance dancing. Life is a dance, and when we dance, we celebrate life as well as exercise the whole body. Dance has an infinite amount to teach us about meditation, because when we are meditating, we are savoring the dance of life on its subtle levels.

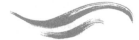

The Emotional Body Scan

Meditation is a time to feel, a place and time to be with your feelings in their unedited form. You don't have to control your feelings in meditation because you are not going to act on them and you are not going to tell anyone what they are. In meditation, you are being with your feelings for no purpose other than that they are calling and you are going to pay attention. Usually we are at the mercy of our level of perception of emotions, which day to day doesn't run very deep. In meditation, our emotions are free to intensify or fade away or change into something else altogether as we pay close attention.

In meditation we may find ourselves hating someone, then painfully admit to ourselves that we envy them, then that changes to sorrow, all in a few seconds. Time expands. After being with the sorrow, a sense of a want emerges, a long-neglected yearning. We want that same thing the person we are envying is living—only we gave up on the desire long ago. It's as if some sort of lubricant were squirted on our emotions, so that the interior mechanisms can slide against each other, a well-oiled machine.

When we feel every particle of emotion and let awareness carry the burden, it takes a great load off the body.

A simple form of meditation you may find useful is to sit quietly somewhere safe and notice what you are feeling. You might ask yourself, "Hmm, what am I feeling?" or you could wonder wordlessly. Be aware of your overall emotional tone, and also whatever sensations you have in your body that seem related to emotion. The heart area, the throat, the belly, the pelvis, the arms, the face—all have subtly different ways of registering emotional sensation. Some areas will feel needy; allow your attention to be called there.

Over time you will notice a correlation between sensations or aches you may feel in your body, and emotions that seem trapped, condensed, or active in that body part. Everyone has a different map, an individual way he channels emotion through the body. Emotions want to be in motion, they want to flow through you and out into the world. When expression is stymied, we can ache simply from the lack of expression.

LORIN'S NOTEBOOK

JACK: THE MAGIC OF MEDITATION

Jack is a theoretical physicist who sings opera on the side. He is attracted to strong passion, but his conscious self is extremely intellectual. At one time, when he was feeling emotions he tended to injure himself while playing tennis, or shaving, or walking, or he would get intense colds that would last a long time.

When Jack began meditating, he cried, laughed, shouted, shook, and vibrated for months. All the emotions that were pent up came out. Sometimes he would sit, shaking or shuddering, for a half-hour at a time. Afterward he would feel brand new, lighter and younger than he had in years. It took almost a year for this dramatic (well, in the context of meditation) catharsis to be fulfilled. Then meditating became mostly a smooth release for a year or so.

After several years of meditation, Jack looked physically different. His habitual scientist's scowl gave way to a relaxed, amused expression. Now he dances, sings, and takes long walks frequently. His whole world has opened up, as they say. Even though he spends far less time at work, he gets more done, publishing twice as many papers as before. For Jack, meditation worked powerful magic.

Here you can see another realm of the play of opposites in meditation, because finding satisfying and ethical ways to fully express your emotions leads to clearer and deeper meditations. And deep meditation leads to contact with your inner life, which leads to further impulses to express yourself. Meditation and expression are complementary opposites.

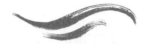

The Instincts and the Daily Body Scan

As you begin to sense what you need, you may find that being aware of the instincts puts you into a resourceful state. Sometimes when we are paying attention to the emotional areas of the body, they just seem like endless aching needs. How can you give yourself what you need? Where can you go to get whatever magic stuff they want?

The instincts are richly varied and serve to remind us of what utterly different textures of attention you can give yourself. Many times, it is not enough to just pay attention to aching needs. We need to give ourselves very specific types of attention. Whenever you feel yourself at this kind of a juncture, run through the instincts in your mind, perhaps by thinking the name of each: hunting, homing, nesting, bonding, protecting, feeding, exploring, playing, communicating.

It may take only a moment to activate your instincts, to remind yourself of their existence. The brain works very rapidly, and the instincts are hardwired into your nervous system.

Touch every instinct and allow it to function in your life and in meditation.

Notice where in your body you feel each instinct most intensely. Perhaps one instinct makes you extremely aware of your entire skin. Or of being poised in a certain way. Where in your body do you feel sensations, motion, or action potential when you are in this instinctive mode?

What is the direction of motion? Up in the body, out toward the world, down into the lower body or the earth? What is the choreography? In and around, as in a chuckle that you savor before sharing the joke?

- **Enter the parts of the body activated or related to each instinct.**
- **Feel the sensations there.**
- **Breathe with that center.**
- **From there, relate to everywhere else in the body: above, below, front, back.**
- **Go in to the center.**
- **Relate the center to the world.**
- **Dissolve the center into your entire body.**
- **Dissolve your entire body into the world.**
- **Rest attention in some sweet spot inside yourself.**
- **Relate from there to the entire body.**

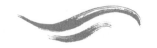

Minute Meditations

In addition to your daily body scan, here are some quick meditations you can grab throughout the day. Each one takes a minute or less and can be done almost anywhere. A minute can make a huge difference in how you feel. Find the ones that work best for you, and adapt them freely to your needs. In so doing, you will build skills that help you with longer meditations. Or you can start out with one or more of these when you are beginning a longer meditation session and then just extend the time.

You won't go very deep into meditation with the following, but this is desirable. You can practice the skills you need to ride your rhythms, and get used to just letting your nervous system shift a little bit into healing mode.

Take a conscious breath: Take a breather. Put your attention on the flow of breath as it comes in through the nose, swirls around in the sinuses, glides down the throat, and fills the lungs. The whole torso expands and contracts with each breath. Each time you do this you can find new sensations to enjoy.

Attitude of gratitude: Call to mind something you are grateful for, then take one conscious breath to savor the feeling while you touch your fingertips to the center of your chest.

Listen with your whole body: If someone is talking to you, give them all the attention they are asking for. Let them be the center of the universe.

The instant mental vacation: Imagine yourself anywhere you'd rather be right now: in Tahiti, at a ballgame, in bed with your lover, wherever. What colors do you see, what sounds do you hear, how does the air smell in that place? Take a few conscious breaths in the spirit of that enjoyment. Savor the feeling of being away from it all. Notice the relief you feel, how your muscles relax, your skin feels soothed, your eyes can stop squinting.

Tai chi breath: Let your hands float in front of you. Inhale slowly, drawing your palms inward toward your chest. As you exhale, turn the palms and let them glide back out. The slower the movement, the more relaxing this is.

Passion: Anytime you find yourself in a moment of passion, pause, celebrate the feeling, and say to yourself, *I am.*

Energizer breath: Sit or stand and breathe rapidly in and out through the nose, the way you would when walking at a brisk clip. Or you can pant as during sex. Do this for 30 seconds, then pause. If you enjoy the sensations, then do another 30 seconds.

The instant nap: Close your eyes and pretend you are taking a nap. Let your muscles start to relax—they know how—in the same way as when you fall asleep. This is a power nap, and even a couple of minutes are restorative. You may daydream, fantasize, or nod off for a minute. When you open your eyes, move slowly for about 10 seconds in order to reorient yourself.

The slump: Sitting comfortably, let your head droop forward slightly. Feel how gravity pulls you down. Let your chin drop toward your chest and then continue downward however far is comfortable. In the process, relax the shoulders and let them slump. Move slowly enough that you can enjoy the sensations of stretching. Then very slowly straighten your spine and let your head come to the vertical position. Notice any pleasurable sensations.

Exhale slowly: Take a deep breath and exhale as slowly as you can, letting the breath make a whispered *whoo, whew,* or *hoo* sound.

Inhale and hold a breath: Inhale in an easy, natural way, then pause to enjoy the sensation of fullness before exhaling. This can create an almost instant sense of relaxation. Play with the length of time you pause, from a second to several seconds.

Tense and relax: Gently tense any area of your body—your face, shoulders, arms, legs, or butt—and hold the contraction for a few seconds. Then let go and savor the feeling of relaxation. If you have more time, go through your entire body, tensing and letting go and witnessing the luxurious sensations that result.

Center yourself: Standing or sitting, lean slightly to one side and then the other. Then sway forward and back. Notice the pleasure of swaying, then of being upright and still. The movements do not have to be visually apparent to other people. You can literally feel your center of gravity.

Discover slow: When walking, slow down a bit and notice what happens to your sensory experience. Let all your senses open up—look around, use your peripheral vision, listen, smell the air (unless it's filled with exhaust fumes), notice the temperature and humidity of the air. Just by adding a bit of leisure to your gait, you may find that you learn things about your world you didn't notice before.

Just say no: Occasionally you may have the feeling of being invaded by the world. Despite your best efforts at work or home, the pressure just won't let up. Sometimes this irritation can trigger the stress response and lead to a skin rash; the skin is a boundary, and the feeling is that your boundaries are being invaded. Wherever you are when you become aware of feeling itchy and irritated, say *No!* inside of yourself, and even out loud. Give yourself the right to say no to the world and to everything that bothers you. At first, do this for 5 to 10 seconds, just one breath, to see if you can get away with it.

Give yourself space: As you move through the world, give yourself little bits of extra space wherever you are. Keep your distance physically from other people. If you are in line at an ATM or at the market checkout, stand farther back. Even if it is only a couple of inches, you are taking control of the space around you. If you are driving, allow more space between your car and those around you. If you are going to the movies, pick a seat away from the crowd. If you are indoors and circumstances permit, go outdoors and let your attention expand. Focus on the far horizon.

Lost in space: Go somewhere that you can lie on your back and look at the sky, day or at night. It could be on a rooftop, at the beach, on a hill, in your backyard, or in the bed of a pickup truck. Look up and let yourself dissolve into infinity. If you can't lie down, at least look up.

To hell with everyone: Due to the incessant needs and demands of everyday life, your own inner needs are often pushed to the background, sometimes for a long, long time. This creates a feeling of resentment or anger, which then has to be suppressed, and thus you are at war with yourself—a drain to the body and the soul.

There are times, however, when you can take your own side, and this may feel extremely antisocial. Usually the only time responsible people will be in the to-hell-with-everyone state is when they are drunk. But in meditation, you can enter this feeling for just long enough to let your body revel in it. Sometime when you have a minute, close your eyes and think the words inside yourself: *to hell with everyone.* It may feel horrible at first, but then you may see some humor in it. Or, if you want, you may change the words to say something similar.

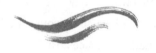

Cultivate Safety

Whether you allow meditation to be deeply healing for you depends on whether you feel emotionally safe enough to tolerate this process. What does safety feel like, and where does it come from? There's a different answer for everyone. For some people it comes from men in white coats (or white, black, or purple robes). They want a doctor or the right kind of guru to authoritatively tell them what to do. If someone wearing the right robes or headdress tells them it's okay to meditate, they'll do it. Other people know from their own experiences with love and life's losses that it is okay to grieve and get over things, and a hell of a lot better than keeping everything corked up inside. Others still have learned this skill in therapy, theater, or dance, and bring that expertise to their meditation and thus have no problem with emotional release.

I once worked with a woman who had left a spiritual center where the teaching and the technique were exactly what she needed and the teacher was brilliant. She went to study at a center where the teacher was a dork and the teaching seemed hokey,

TRAVEL YOUR OWN PATH

Once you have developed a whole body meditation practice that works for you, you may want to avoid talking about your experiences with people who are doing orthodox meditation practices. Their authoritarian attitudes can be as parochial as those of any narrow-minded religion—"Your technique is not meditation; you must bow down to my guru and give him your money; the sacred tradition I practice is the only true form of meditation . . ." —and should not be allowed to compromise your natural instinct to meditate and heal.

The big secret is that there is no secret at all—you will get benefits if you enjoy something in a very natural way. Don't merely concentrate on meditation or bore yourself with it—find out what is interesting about it for you and cultivate your ability to be entertained by the subtle actions of breath and sound (vibration). This is the kind of foundation you want to give yourself in your approach to whole body meditation.

but she had a lot of good friends there. There was a circle of strong, wonderful women there, and that was where she felt safe enough to go through her spiritual and emotional processing.

You can also teach yourself to feel safe by meditating in small increments, 5 or 10 minutes at a time, and checking out how you feel during and after. If you find that you can handle the little bits of emotional release you get and that you feel better afterward, then increase the length of time you spend meditating, up to 20 minutes or so.

Catharsis doesn't always mean crying or being angry during your meditation. Lots of people laugh for months after beginning meditation. They laugh during meditation and afterward. They laugh at the sky, at the sun, and at themselves—what a joke, that they had been taking life so seriously and feeling tyrannized by such tiny things.

One of my friends has a great laugh, and I remarked on it one day. She said, "I started meditating and I started laughing, and look at me, 30 years later I'm still at it—both of 'em."

Sources, Resources,
and Further Explorations

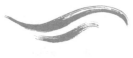

Sources

The Florence Nightingale quote on the epigraph page is from her *Notes on Nursing: What It Is and What It Is Not*, published in 1992 by Lippincott Williams & Wilkins Publishers, pages 74–75. This book was first printed in 1859 and is still in print today. Here is the full quote:

> *It is often thought that medicine is the curative process. It is no such thing; medicine is the surgery of functions, as surgery proper is that of limbs and organs. Nei-*

ther can do anything but remove obstructions; neither can cure; nature alone cures. Surgery removes the bullet out of the limb, which is an obstruction to cure, but nature heals the wound. So it is with medicine; the function of an organ becomes obstructed; medicine, so far as we know, assists nature to remove the obstruction, but does nothing more. And what nursing has to do in either case, is to put the patient in the best condition for nature to act upon him.

Thanks to Helen Sellars of the Florence Nightingale Museum in London for her help in verifying the quote.

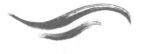

Resources

For word definitions, I always turn first to the sublime *American Heritage Dictionary of the English Language,* published by Houghton Mifflin Company.

For example, with the word *taboo,* the AH gives not only the definition, "A ban or an inhibition resulting from social custom or emotional aversion," but the word history, detailing how Captain James Cook heard the word while exploring the Friendly Islands (Tonga). Cook loved the word and brought it back to England, where it gradually became part of the English language.

Sometimes I use the bound-book version of *American Heritage Dictionary* (fourth edition, 2000), sometimes I access the CD-ROM, and often I look at Web sites that link to the electronic version. During the time I was writing *Whole Body Meditations*, I accessed the dictionary online at www.Bartleby.com. Poking around their site, I found this note from Steven H. van Leeuwen, publisher and founder: "Bartleby.com began as a personal research experiment in 1993 and within one year published the first classic book on the Web (Walt Whitman's *Leaves of Grass*)."

As background literature on self-renewal, I enjoyed reading *Healers on Healing*, edited by Richard Carlson, Ph.D., and Benjamin Shield. The book was published in 1989 by Jeremy Tarcher and consists of brief essays by shaman types, healers, doctors, and meditation teachers.

In "The Taboo against Rest" on page 38, I mention ultradian rhythms, the natural biological rhythms that occur more than once a day (circadian rhythms are those that occur about once a day). Here I am referring to the work of Ernest Lawrence Rossi, Ph.D., whose research applies to all human activities, whether we are meditating, working, or traveling. Dr. Rossi has published many books and articles; one of the most accessible is *The 20 Minute Break*, published in 1991 by Jeremy Tarcher.

When I'm writing, music is my elixir. The way a singer shapes her throat, opens her heart to make a note; the definitive way a drummer lays down a track; and the way a guitarist enters the silence with a chord, a chord that is simultaneously plea, prayer, and assertion, these can revive me and remind me of what life is.

Here is a list of what I listened to most while writing *Whole Body Meditations*:

Herbie Mann and Joao Gilberto, *Deve Ser Amor*

Sade, *King of Sorrow, Immigrant*

Enigma, *Beyond the Invisible, Silent Warrior*

Van Morrison, *Shenandoah, Have I Told You Lately*

David Parsons, *Parikrama*

Nick Drake, *Cello Song*

Tommy Dorsey, *Moonlight in Vermont*

Astrud Gilberto and Gil Evans, *I Will Wait for You*

Joao Gilberto, *'s Wonderful*

Jennifer Warnes and Leonard Cohen, *Joan of Arc*

Artie Shaw, *Deep Purple*

Crosby, Stills and Nash, *Wooden Ships*

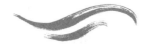

Further Explorations

I don't know why there is not more discussion of the mythic cycle as it pertains to moment-by-moment experience in meditation. It is such a useful tool for understanding what happens every 15 seconds or so in meditation.

I highly recommend reading Joseph Campbell's *The Hero with a Thousand Faces*, published in 1968 by Princeton University Press. Campbell takes you on a tour of the world's myths and fairy tales, showing the similar plot structures: the call to adventure, meeting with helpers, the threshold crossing, tests, then the elixir theft (or Sacred Marriage or meeting with God), followed by perhaps a struggle to return to the land of everyday and, finally, the return.

THWTF, as it is called by some, is enchanting reading. The book was assigned reading for a class I took in early 1968, and I read it every day for about an hour, at 4 in the morning while sitting in the bath and at the beach between waves. Over the next year, I probably read it cover to cover several dozen times.

Campbell's ideas have been disseminated far and wide. In the movie business, George Lucas apparently consulted *THWTF* when writing the scripts for his *Star Wars* movies. Writer Christopher Vogler has taken Campbell's ideas and uses scenes from popular movies such as *The Wizard of Oz*, *The Full Monty*, *Pulp Fiction*, *The Lion King*, and *Titanic*, to name a few, to illustrate the phases of the mythic journey. Vogler's book *The Writer's Journey: Mythic Structure for Writers*, published in 1998 by Michael Wiese Productions, is not just for writers; I think it is a great teaching book. Another book on the mythic structure of movies is Stuart Voytilla's *Myth and the Movies: Discovering the Mythic Structure of 50 Unforgettable Films*, also published by Wiese.

Knowing the plot structure does not take anything away from being enchanted by a story, myth, or fairy tale. If anything, this knowledge heightens the appreciation, since your brain uses the same narrative structure every night when you dream. The brain loves a story.

~

On the evolution of meditation techniques: We are in an extraordinarily fecund period, where new combinations of meditation instructions are emerging daily. Everyone is borrowing or stealing from everyone else, often without knowing it or knowing the source. Of course, the basic ideas are ancient, but the combinations are like cooking styles—there is always something fresh you can do. Buddhist techniques are being changed into Christian contemplations; Jungians can rightfully claim that everyone is using their Active Imagination techniques out of context; hypnosis, massage, and the latest brain research are being combined and presented as a new form of meditation. The purists scream about "the purity of the teaching," and yet this atmosphere of recombination and free-ranging exploration is exactly what gave rise to the spiritual riches of ancient India, China, and Tibet, of course.

I have been enjoying some of the guided meditations put out by the Mind/Body Medical Institute at Harvard. Although they call it meditation, the imagery they use is that of hypnosis and the people who developed self-hypnotism. Hypnotists, especially those trained in neurolinguistic programming (NLP), tend to be excellent with language, very evocative. They really work at it. (Connirae and Steve Andreas do a brilliant job of making the NLP insights accessible. NLP is itself based on the work of three geniuses: Fritz Perls's Gestalt therapy, Virginia Satir's work with families and couples, and Milton Erickson's practice of hypnotherapy. Each has spawned a huge literature.) Those involved with defining the Guided Imagery and Music method, which is now being used with cancer and Alzheimer patients, among others, did pioneering work in developing this approach.

❧

To get your own sense of the field of words, log on to www.VisualThesaurus.com. Set the program to 3-D and autonavigate, put on your favorite music, and type in a word that you are interested in. You'll learn something about semantics, the dancing interconnectedness of words that's so vividly illustrated here.

❧

T. S. Eliot evokes the Taboo against Aliveness (see page 40) in *The Love Song of J. Alfred Prufrock* (1915): "Do I dare / Disturb the universe?"

❧

If your concern is pain caused by physical injury to muscles, bones, tendons, or joints, I recommend *Listen to Your Pain: The Active Person's Guide to Understanding, Identifying, and Treating Pain and Injury* by Ben Benjamin, Ph.D., with Gale Borden, M.D., published in 1984 by Penguin Books.

❧

I loved reading *The Powerful Placebo: From Ancient Priest to Modern Physician* by Arthur K. Shapiro, M.D., and Elaine Shapiro, Ph.D., published in 1997 by Johns

Hopkins University Press. This wife-and-husband team has done a magnificent job of bringing together a history of the placebo effect in ancient India, Greece, Babylon, China, and Rome. If you are taking herbs or going to health food stores for vitamins and supplements, you should read this book. The Shapiros worked long and thought deeply on the subject, and the book is full of subtlety and interesting asides. Consider this comment, in a discussion of how to do research on the effects of psychotherapy: "While the use of standardized psychotherapeutic manuals is praiseworthy, to an unknown extent they deprive psychotherapists of their spontaneity, sensitivity, flexibility, warmth, genuineness, empathy, ability to resourcefully respond to unpredictable and idiosyncratic situations, and adequate motivation for effective psychotherapy. . . . Psychotherapists may feel like dull-witted clods, dispensing fortune-cookie advice, maxims, and predictions" (from page 116).

❧

A good introduction to the instincts is *The Three Faces of Mind* by Elaine de Beauport with Aura Sofia Diaz, published in 1996 by Quest Books. These two brilliant thinkers come at the instincts through brain structure, and the book is extremely readable and full of explorations and meditations.

To get a sense of how instinctive variety is seamlessly woven into meditation texts, look at the 11th step in *Twelve Steps and Twelve Traditions*, the AA guidebook. Also, in the *The Long Road Turns to Joy*, Thich Nhat Hanh recommends instinctive richness when doing Vipassana meditation.

❧

There are many places you can go to learn about the meditative sense of hunting. To get inside the head of a tracker, read Tom Brown Jr.'s *Awakening Spirits*, published in 1994. Laurens van der Post has written extensively about hunting in Africa, with the sensibility of a Jungian analyst. Arnold Mindell's *The Shaman's Body*, published in 1993 by HarperSanFrancisco, is a description of the hunting instinct as it shows up in modern-day shamanism.

❧

I highly recommend *The Erotic Silence of the American Wife* by Dalma Heyn, published in 1997 by Penguin Books. I don't know why this book is not immensely famous. It is women talking about what they crave in sex, and the intimacy they long for that sometimes drives them to have extramarital affairs.

One of my meditation students told me about this book. She married her high school sweetheart, and after 25 years of marriage she found herself totally alive and in love with her husband, but also neglected and expected to play only the roles of mother, cook, maid, chauffeur, showpiece, and homework helper in their tiny Midwestern town. She was restless and desperately trying not to have an extramarital affair, even though her entire world was conspiring to lead her there.

What Heyn has an ear for is the sensual, bodily experience of being free to love—what you feel like in the midst of your day just because you have the possibility of being able to let your love flow freely with a new person. Meditation often feels this way, like having an affair, because there is the possibility of falling in love with life, and this feels slightly illicit. In meditation, the situation is not outer. There is no outer person. It has to do with your inner circuits. Why shouldn't you be erotically in love with life, breath, gravity? You run across the taboos just the same as if you were having an outer relationship, and you must negotiate your own way through what works in your life. How much sexual aliveness can you tolerate?

~

Every human being in Western civilization should read *Why Zebras Don't Get Ulcers: An Updated Guide to Stress, Stress-Related Disorders, and Coping* by Robert M. Sapolsky, published in 1998 by W. H. Freeman and Company. Sapolsky is just the best at describing the physical effects of both temporary and chronic stress, and his lively mind makes the reading very entertaining.

~

For more information on the physiology of meditation, you can't do better than reading Benson himself—Dr. Herbert Benson, the cardiologist from Harvard who has been doing research on the physiology of meditation since the late 1960s. I recommend his *Timeless Healing: The Power and Biology of Belief,* published in 1996 by Scribner.

Index

Underscored page references indicate boxed text. **Boldface** references indicate illustrations.

A

AA 12-step program, x, 104–5
Adaptability, 63, 70
Adaptations, 33
Addictions, 33
Adventure of meditation, 124
Air element, 128–30, 129
Alcoholics Anonymous 12-step program, x, 104–5
Aliveness taboo, 40–41
Allies, instinct, 68–69
Alternative health movement, 83, 119, 123–24
Anahata chakra, 160
Answering the call, 25
Approach to meditation, recommended, xvi–xvii
Arms meditations, 184–85
Arms scan, 182, 184–85
Attention, 111–17
    body parts and, 63–64
    going beyond, 160–61
    instincts, 14
    loving and, xvii

in meditation, 109–11
pain and, 117–19, 118, 120–21, 122–23

B

Back meditations, 202–3
Balance experiences, 56
Belly breath meditation, 198–99
Belly meditations, 198–200
Belly scan, 197–200
Benson, Dr. Herbert, 50
Biofeedback methods, 153
Blame, avoiding self, 156–58
Blessing hands meditation, 185
Body
    attention to parts of, 63–64
    bones, 206
    circulation, 206
    dancing and, 207
    dimensions of, 206–8
    elements of, 59–60
    immune system, 206
    listening with whole, 214

Body *(cont.)*
  nervous system, 207
  questioning, <u>180</u>
  rebuilding, 60–62
  reinhabiting, 10–13, <u>11</u>
  skin, 206
  space, 207
  strangulation of parts of, <u>199</u>
  synchronization of, <u>61</u>
  whole body salute and, 207
Body scan, 179, 181
  abandoning, 11
  arms, 182, 184–85
  belly, lower, 197–200
  chest, 192–95
  dimensions of body and, 206–8
  emotional, 208–11
  eyes, <u>190–91</u>
  feet, 186–88
  hands, 182, 184–85
  head, 188–92
  instincts and, 211–13
  legs, 186–88
  map, **183**
  minute meditations with, 213–17
  mouth, <u>191</u>
  neck, 203–5
  pelvis, 197–200
  questioning the body and, <u>180</u>
  results of, 179, 181–82
  safety and, 217–19
  solar plexus, 195–97
  spine, 200–203
  strangulation and, <u>199</u>
  throat, 203–4, <u>204–5</u>
Bones, 206
Boundaries
  changing, <u>125</u>
  crossing, <u>90</u>

Bowel purification, 82–84, <u>83</u>
Breathing
  belly, 198–99
  chanting and, 140
  conscious, 213
  diaphragmatic, 196
  energizer, 214
  exhaling, 82, 215
  with feet and legs meditation, 188
  flow of, 56
  and humming meditation, 192
  inhaling, 215
  palate, 190
  pulsing, 197
  tai chi, 214
  wonderment and, <u>71</u>
  yoga, 84
Breath Taking (Roche), 32

C

Caduceus meditations, 201–2
Call to meditation, <u>14</u>, 16–18, <u>161</u>
Calming space meditation, 185
Centering self, 215
Chanting, 125, 140, 199–200
Cherish your heartbeat meditation, 193–94
Chest meditations, 193–95
Chest scan, 192–95
Chi gung, 80
Christian approach to meditation, 105–6
Circulation, 206
Coaching for meditation, xiv–xv, <u>126</u>, <u>152–53</u>.
    See also Guides; Teachers
Communication instinct, 69, 92–93
Community, 90–92
Complementary medicine, meditation as, <u>119</u>
Counseling, <u>46</u>, 49
Crossing boundaries instinct, <u>90</u>
Crossing thresholds, 19, 24–25

Cultlike meditation groups, <u>126</u>
Cycles of meditation, 75, 169–72

D

Dancing, 207–8, <u>208</u>
Death, 49
Denying instincts, <u>101</u>
Depression, 46, 48–49
Descent taboo, 45–46, 48–50
Diaphragmatic breathing meditation, 196
Dimensions of body, 206–8
Disabilities, 46, 48
Discovery, 215

E

Earth element, 130–32, <u>131</u>
Electroencephalogram (EEG), <u>153</u>
Electromyogram (EMG), <u>153</u>
Elements. *See also* Explorations of elements
   air, 128–30, <u>129</u>
   alternative medicine and, 123–24
   of body, 59–60
   earth, 130–32, <u>131</u>
   familiarizing yourself with, 124–25, 127–28
   fire, 132–35, <u>133</u>
   focusing on, 143
   imagery and, 125–27
   space, 135–36, <u>135</u>
   vibration, 137–40, <u>137</u>
   water, 140–42
Elixirs
   meditation as, 30
   reaching for, 27–31, <u>28–29</u>
   of whole body meditation, 12–13
Emergency stress response, 35–36
EMG, <u>153</u>
Emotional body scan, 208–11
Emotional effects of meditation, 112–13,
   <u>170</u>

Emotions, controlling, 44
Energizer breathing, 214
Essence of meditation, xvii
Excretion instinct, 82–84, <u>83</u>
Exhaling breath, 82, 215
Explorations of elements
   air, 129, <u>129</u>
   earth, 132
   fire, 134
   space, 136
   vibration, 140
   water, 141
Exploring instinct, 71–72, <u>71</u>
Eyes scan, <u>190–91</u>

F

Feelings of meditation, 169–72, <u>170</u>
Feet meditations, 187–88
Feet scan, 186–88
Fire element, 132–35, <u>133</u>
Flow of breath experiences, 56
Forging alliances, 98–100
Format, standard meditative, <u>147</u>
Franklin, Benjamin, 129
Fulfilling journey, <u>54–55</u>

G

Galvanic skin response monitoring device
   (GSR), <u>153</u>
Gathering instinct, 79–81, <u>79</u>
God instinct, 96–98
Gratitude, attitude of, 213
Gravity, <u>131</u>
Grooming instinct, 69, 76–77
GSR, <u>153</u>
Guardians, threshold, 37
Guides, xiv–xv, <u>126</u>
Guilt, <u>47</u>
Gut responses, <u>88</u>

H

Hands meditations, 184–85
Hands scan, 182, 184–85
Hands to head meditation, 192
Hanh, Thich Nhat, 106
Headaches, 123
Head meditations, 189–92
Head scan, 188–92
Healing. *See also* Self-healing
  cycle
    answering the call, 25
    bringing it home, 31–32
    crossing thresholds, 19, 24–25
    example of, 122
    initiating to self, 25–27
    mythic cycle and, 15–16
    reaching for elixir, 27–31, 28–29
    refusing the call, 18–19, 20–23
    rhythm of, 17, 18
    symptoms as callings, 16–18
  instincts, 11–12
  memory and, 48
  quest for wholeness and, 7–10
    sensual experience of, 53, 56–57
  rest and, 38–39
  spontaneous, 42
Heartbeat, 193–94
Heart meditation technique, 160
Herding instinct, 90–92
Hinduism, 106
Ho-ho-ho meditation, 199–200
Homing instinct, 72–74, 73
Humming and breathing meditation, 192
Hunting instinct, 77–79

I

Illness, xi, 7, 10
Imagery, 11, 125–27, 214
Imagination, 85–86, 85

Immune system, 206
Individuality in meditation, 150–56, 167–68
Inhaling breath, 215
Initiation to self, 13–15, 14, 25–27
Inner movement experiences, 56
Inner power, 62–66
Instincts
  allies of, journeying with, 68–69
  attention, 14
  being in touch with all, 79
  body scan and, 211–13
  body's elements and, 59–60
  communication, 69, 92–93
  crossing boundaries, 90
  crossing thresholds and accessing, 24
  denying, 101
  excretion, 82–84, 83
  exploring, 71–72, 71
  following, 66–68
  forging alliances and, 98–100
  gathering, 79–81, 79
  God, 96–98
  grooming, 69, 76–77
  healing, 11–12
  herding, 90–92
  homing, 72–74, 73
  hunting, 77–79
  inner power and, 62–66
  loving, 93–96, 94
  meditating, xvi, 65
  nurturing, 70, 81–82
  overcoming obstacles to, 102–3
  play, 84–86, 85
  problems with, 100–103, 101, 102–3
  protecting, 69, 86–90, 87, 88
  quest for wholeness and, 69–70
  rebuilding body and, 60–62
  reclaiming, 15
  rest, 69, 74–76, 75

in sacred traditions, 104–7, <u>105</u>
tone and, 144
Instructions for meditation, xiv, 142–45, <u>145</u>
Internal guidance, <u>126</u>

J

Journey fulfilled, <u>54–55</u>
Joy to the world meditation, 194
Jung, Carl, 19

K

King, Martin Luther Jr., 106

L

Language, 137–40, <u>137</u>, 138–39
Legs meditations, 187–88
Legs scan, 186–88
Letting go, <u>75</u>
Life
    rhythm of, ix–x, 3–4, 74
    vital, 70
Lighten up meditation, 189
Light experiences, 53, <u>75</u>, <u>133</u>
Listening
    learning and, <u>67</u>
    with whole body, 214
Listening to heart meditation, 194
Long Road Turns to Joy, The (Hanh), 106
Loving
    attention and, xvii
    instinct, 93–96, <u>94</u>
    meditation as, <u>94</u>
    touch, <u>90</u>

M

Magnetic hands meditation, 184–85
Mantras, 125, 140, 199–200
Map, body scan, **183**
Map-firsters, 45

Martial arts, <u>87</u>
Maslow, Abraham, <u>79</u>
Medicine
    alternative, <u>83</u>, 123–24
    meditation as complementary, <u>119</u>
    root word of, 109
Memory and healing, <u>48</u>
Mental effects of meditation, 115–17
Mind-body system, ix, 63
Mindfulness concept, <u>148</u>
Minute meditations, 213–17
"Monkey mind," managing, <u>164–65</u>
Mouth scan, <u>191</u>
Moving the world meditation, 187
Mythic cycle, <u>6</u>, 15–16
Mythic journey, 6, <u>8–9</u>, <u>11</u>

N

Nap, instant, 214
Neck scan, 203–5
Nervous system, 207
Notice your inner theater meditation, 189
Nurturing instinct, 70, 81–82

O

Obstacles to meditation
    common sense and, <u>161</u>, 163
    following your heart and, <u>160–61</u>
    individuality and, 167–68
    mental weapons in countering, <u>164–65</u>
    "monkey mind," <u>164–65</u>
    pain and, 166–67
    personal experiences, 158–59, 162
    teachers and guides and, 162–63
    unmet needs and, 163–66
Opportunity, 13–14
Orthodox meditation, 218
Outer life, meditation's effects on, 31–32
Overcoming obstacles, <u>102–3</u>

P

Pain
  accepting, 26–27
  attention and, 117–19, <u>118</u>, <u>120–21</u>, 122–23
  being with, 117–19, <u>118</u>, <u>120–21</u>, 122–23
  calling of, 11, 117
  headaches, 123
  levels, <u>120–21</u>
  meditation and, 52–53
  motivation of, 12
  as obstacle to meditation, 166–67
  responses to, 16
Palate breathing meditation, 190
Passion, 214
Pelvis meditations, 198–99
Pelvis scan, 197–200
Personal experiences with meditation
  eyes scan, <u>190–91</u>
  journey fulfilled, <u>54–55</u>
  magic of meditation, <u>210</u>
  mouth scan, <u>191</u>
  obstacles to meditation, 158–59, 162
  overcoming obstacles, <u>102–3</u>
  pain levels, <u>120–21</u>
  reaching for elixir, <u>28–29</u>
  refusing the call, <u>20–23</u>
  regrets, <u>47</u>
  remembering wellness, <u>51</u>
  resources for meditation, <u>145</u>
  spontaneous healing, <u>42</u>
  throat meditation, <u>204–5</u>
  vacation from meditation, <u>154–55</u>
Physical effects of meditation, x–xi, <u>5</u>, 35,
      113–15, <u>114</u>
Placebo effect, 50–52
Planted firmly in the ground meditation, 187
Play instinct, 84–86, <u>85</u>
Pleasure taboo, 39–40
Power within, 62–66

Pranayama, 84
Process of meditation, 125, 157–58
  attention and, 111–17
  emotional effects, 112–13
  feelings about, 169–72, <u>170</u>
  instructions, xiv, 142–45, <u>145</u>
  mental effects, 115–17
  orthodox, 218
  physical effects, x–ix, <u>5</u>, 113–15, <u>114</u>
  research on, 111
  simplicity and, 146, 148–49
Protecting instinct, 69, 86–90, <u>87</u>, <u>88</u>
Psychic callus, 163–64
Pulsing breathing meditation, 197

Q

Quest for wholeness
  crossing thresholds and, 24
  healing and, 7–10
    sensual experience of, 53, 56–57
  healing cycle and
    answering the call, 25
    bringing it home, 31–32
    crossing thresholds, 19, 24–25
    example of, 122
    initiating to self, 25–27
    mythic cycle and, 15–16
    reaching for elixir, 27–31, <u>28–29</u>
    refusing the call, 18–19, <u>20–23</u>
    rhythm of, <u>17</u>, 18
    symptoms as callings and, 16–18
  initiation to self and, 13–15, <u>14</u>,
      25–27
  instincts and, 69–70
  meditation and, 99
  mythic journey and, 6, <u>8–9</u>, <u>11</u>
  reinhabiting the body and, 10–13, <u>11</u>
  remembering wellness and, 50–53, <u>51</u>
  stress and, 32–36, <u>34</u>

taboos
  aliveness, 40–41
  confronting, 37–38
  descent, 45–46, 48–50
  pleasure, 39–40
  rest, 38–39
  self-care, 37
  spontaneity, 41, 43–45
Questioning the body, <u>180</u>

R

Rebuilding the body, 60–62
Refusing the call, 18–19, <u>20–23</u>
Regrets, <u>47</u>
Reinhabiting the body, 10–13, <u>11</u>
Relaxation
  meditation and, 35–36
  safety and, <u>87</u>
  stress and, xi, 117, 215
Relaxation Response, The (Benson), 50
Religion, 96–98, 105–6
Remembering wellness, 50–53, <u>51</u>
Resources on meditation, xiv, <u>145</u>
Rest
  healing and, 38–39
  instinct, 69, 74–76, <u>75</u>
  nap and, instant, 214
  rebuilding body and, 60–62
  taboo, 38–39
Rest/activation cycle in meditation, 169–72
Rhythm
  of healing cycle, **17**, 18
  of life, ix–x, 3–4, 74
  of meditation, xi–xiii, 4, 122, 172–73, **174**, 175–76
Rock your pelvis meditation, 198

S

Sacred context, finding, <u>105</u>, 106
Sacred traditions, 104–7, <u>105</u>

Safety
  body scan and, 217–19
  cultivating sense of, 26
  meditation and, <u>87</u>
  relaxation and, <u>87</u>
Saying "no," 216
Secret longing meditations, 185, 195
Self-blame, avoiding, 156–58
Self-care taboo, 37
Self-coaching, <u>152–53</u>
Self-healing, x, <u>5</u>
  capacity for, ix
  individuality in, xv–xvi
  placebo effect and, 52
Self-help groups, x, 104–5
Self-nurturing, 81
Sense, focusing on, 143–44
Simple fullness concept, <u>148</u>
Simplicity, returning to, 146, 148–49
Skill of meditation, xvi
Skin, 206
Sleep taboo, 38–39
Slowing motion of head meditation, 191
Slumping, 214–15
Solar plexus meditations, 196–97
Solar plexus scan, 195–97
Sound experiences, 53, 137–40, <u>137</u>, 138–39
Space
  body, 207
  calming, 185
  element of, 135–36, <u>135</u>
  giving to self, 216
  losing self in, 216
  personal, 216
Speech, 137–40, <u>137</u>, 138–39
Spine meditations, 201–2
Spine scan, 200–203
Spirituality, 96–98, 105–6

Spontaneity taboo, 41, 43–45
Stability, internal, 63
State of meditation, xi–xiii, 7–9, 39, 113
Strangulation of body parts, 199
Stress
    adaptations and, 33
    chronic, xi, 33, 35
    emergency response, 35–36
    everyday, 10
    illness and, xi
    meditation and, 117
    personal responses to, 34
    physical responses to, 34, 35
    quest for wholeness and, 32–36, 34
    rapidity of sloughing off, 114
    relaxation and, xi, 117, 215
Sunlight, 75, 133
Survivors of serious disease, 7
Symptoms as callings, 16–18
Synchronization of body, 61

T

Taboos on quest for wholeness
    aliveness, 40–41
    confronting, 37–38
    descent, 45–46, 48–50
    pleasure, 39–40
    rest, 38–39
    self-care, 37
    spontaneity, 41, 43–45
Tai chi, 80, 214
Teachers, xiv–xv, 126
Techniques, 125, 157–58, 160
Tension. See Stress
Therapy, 46, 49
Thoughts during meditation, 20–21, 26, 43, 173, 175–76
Thresholds
    crossing, 19, 24–25
    guardians of, 37

Throat massage with sound meditation, 204–5
Throat meditations, 203–5, 204–5
Throat relaxer meditation, 203–4, 204–5
Throat scan, 203–5, 204–5
Time for self, 216–17
TM, 150
Tone, instinctive, 144
Top-downers, 45
Touch
    experiences, 56
    inappropriate, 88
    loving, 90
Transcendence, 36
Transcendental meditation (TM), 150

V

Vacation
    from meditation, 154–55
    mental, 214
Vibrate the head with sound meditation, 192
Vibration element, 137–40, 137
Vision and meditation, 176
Visualization, 11, 125–27, 214
Voice, 137–40, 137, 138–39
Vowel sounds, 138–39

W

Water element, 140–42
Wellness
    remembering, 50–53, 51
    as whole body experience, 4
Whole body salute, 207
Wholeness. See Quest for wholeness
Wonderment, 71
Workouts, daily, 61–62

Y

Yawning, 191
Yoga breathing, 84